W9-BWZ-622

WITHDRAWN

Funding for this grant was provided by
the Illinois State Library, a Division of
the Office of Secretary of State, using
federal LSTA funding.

Also by Seymour Diamond, M.D.

The Practicing Physician's Approach to Headache,
1st to fifth edition (with Donald J. Dalessio, M.D.)

The Hormone Headache
(with Bill Still and Cynthia Still)

Headache and Diet: Tyramine-Free Recipes
(with Diane Francis and Amy Diamond Vye)

Diagnosing and Managing Headaches,
1st to 3d edition

Hope for Your Headache Problem:
More Than Two Aspirin (with Amy Diamond Vye)

CONQUERING
YOUR
MIGRAINE

The Essential Guide to Understanding and Treating Migraines for All Sufferers and Their Families

Seymour Diamond, M.D.

with **Mary A. Franklin**

A Fireside Book
Published by Simon & Schuster
New York   London   Toronto   Sydney   Singapore

FIRESIDE
Rockefeller Center
1230 Avenue of the Americas
New York, NY 10020

FIRESIDE and colophon are registered trademarks
of Simon & Schuster, Inc.

Designed by William Ruoto

Manufactured in the United States of America

1   3   5   7   9   10   8   6   4   2

Library of Congress Cataloging-in-Publication Data
Diamond, Seymour, date.
Conquering your migraine : the essential guide to understanding
and treating migraines for all sufferers
and their families / Seymour Diamond, with Mary A. Franklin.
p.   cm.
Includes index.
1. Migraine—Popular works.   I. Franklin, Mary A.   II. Title.
RC392 .D4958 2001
616.8'57—dc21
00-066178

ISBN 0-684-87310-9

ACKNOWLEDGMENTS

We would like to thank Marah Stets for her invaluable editorial assistance and patience in the production of this book. Also, we would like to express our appreciation to Ivy Stone for realizing the needs of the migraine patient and expediting publication of this book.

To the misunderstood, misdiagnosed, and mistreated migraine sufferers throughout the world. To Elaine for her encouragement and sagacity.

S.D.

To my son Tim and to Aunt Imie, for their support and tolerance.

M.A.F.

CONTENTS

PART II: TREATING YOUR MIGRAINE

CONQUERING
YOUR
MIGRAINE

PREFACE

For the past thirty-seven years, I have labored in the field of headache. But how did I enter into this specialty? In my family practice in Chicago, I worked with anti-depressants—doing clinical research before these drugs were marketed. I observed in many of my patients that the antidepressants improved many physical complaints, as well as depression. These drugs seemed to be particularly effective in relieving chronic pain.

In 1963, at a medical conference where I was presenting my work on antidepressants in clinical practice, I was asked an innocuous question by another physician—had I observed a relationship between headache and depression? As I had never considered a connection between these two conditions, that question prompted my future interest and dedication to headache research and treatment.

My interest in headache led me to become an early member, officer, and power behind the growth of the American Association for the Study of Headache (now the

American Headache Society). In 1970, I founded the National Migraine Foundation (now the National Headache Foundation), and remain its executive chairperson. The National Headache Foundation is the premier headache organization for headache sufferers.

Beyond our shores, I also served as executive officer of the World Federation of Neurology Research Group on Headache and Migraine. I have also taught neurology, leading to a professorship at Chicago Medical School, as well as a professorship in family medicine and in molecular biology and pharmacology.

In 1972, I limited my practice to headache patients and established the Diamond Headache Clinic, which is the largest and oldest private headache clinic in the United States. In addition to our outpatient facility, located in the Lincoln Park area of Chicago, I direct the forty-one-bed Diamond Inpatient Headache Unit at Columbus Hospital, an affiliate of Catholic Health Partners in Chicago.

During my career, I have published more than three hundred scientific articles, and have written or coauthored more than twenty books for both the professional and the lay reader. My interest in headache has led me throughout the world lecturing on this topic. I remain in active practice at the Diamond Headache Clinic, and fortunately have time to participate in headache research and promote the education of the public on this malady.

And why this book, *Conquering Your Migraine*? Since there are so many books written about headache, I felt that my hands-on approach to counseling headache patients and working with them through their problems would add an element to this book that differs from other available "headache" texts. In my practice, the most difficult cases are referred to me—from not only within the United States but also throughout the world. I constantly am being asked by practicing physicians as well as resident physicians if I would allow them to spend time at the Diamond Headache Clinic—observing both our outpatient facility and the inpatient unit. I hope that my experiences and practicality in handling headache patients will be helpful in directing the readers to the knowledge they seek.

Also, during the past ten years, there have been marked advances in headache research and treatment. These advances integrated with my personal success in treating headache patients make this book's perspective unique.

—Seymour Diamond, M.D.
Chicago, Illinois

PART I
UNDERSTANDING MIGRAINE

Pain has an element of blank;
It cannot recollect
When it began, or if there were
A day when it was not.
It has no future but itself,
Its infinite realms contain
Its past, enlightened to perceive
New periods of pain.

—EMILY DICKINSON,
"Pain Has an Element of Blank"

CHAPTER 1
What Is Migraine?

Headache is the most common pain known to humans. It has been estimated that as many as 80 million Americans suffer from headaches. For many of us, headache is a minor occurrence that can be relieved by an over-the-counter remedy. However, not all headaches are alike and some may be so frequent and severe that the sufferer cannot perform normal, daily activities.

Noted headache sufferers include Lewis Carroll, Virginia Woolf, Thomas Jefferson, Saint Paul, Calvin, Julius Caesar, Chopin, Tchaikovsky, Darwin, George Bernard Shaw, Karl Marx, and Cervantes. It is refreshing to know that headaches did not prevent the creative spirit of these headache sufferers—in fact, at times the headaches inspired their work. For example, the images found in *Through the Looking Glass*, such as when Alice changes size, are believed to represent the auras suffered by the author, Lewis Carroll.

The focus of this book is one form of headache—

migraine. Approximately 28 million Americans suffer from this disorder. The economic impact of migraine is enormous, with 150 million lost days from work or school in the United States, and $13 billion lost in productivity. The price of medications—both prescribed and over-the-counter—and the costs of repeated physician and emergency department visits are mind-boggling.

We believe that one step on the road to recovery for migraine sufferers is education—knowing what their headache is and how to prevent the repeated attacks. We hope to encourage those with migraine to seek help so that they will not have a life defined by their head pain.

What Is a Migraine?

Before we can understand migraine headaches and their treatment, we must have a clear picture of the major forms of headache. The simplest classification of headaches that we use is divided into three categories—tension-type, organic, and vascular.

Tension-type (muscle contraction) *headaches* are due to the body's reaction to stress, anxiety, depression, emotional conflicts, fatigue, or repressed hostility. Although a certain increase in muscle spasm occurs with tension-type headaches, we now use the term "tension-type" because we believe that some of the provoking factors (stress, tension) may affect the brain's pain centers as well as the localized muscle contractions. The headaches have been described as pressure, tightening, a headband or caplike sensation, or viselike. The pain may present across the forehead, in the temples, or at the back of the head or neck. These headaches are two-sided, and vary from mild to moderate severity. Associated symptoms are uncommon.

Tension-type headaches are further divided into two types—episodic and chronic. We have all suffered the episodic, occasional tension-type headache, which is usually relieved by over-the-counter pain relievers (aspirin, acetaminophen, ibuprofen, naproxen sodium).

The episodic type is easily managed with over-the-counter analgesics, including the nonsteroidal anti-inflammatory drugs (NSAIDs). Anti-inflammatory agents reduce swelling and irritation associated with inflammation throughout the body. This category includes the corticosteroids and the NSAIDs. The NSAIDs are the drugs of choice in treating intermittent or episodic tension-type headaches.

Chronic tension-type headaches are daily or almost-daily continuous headaches, and usually affect both sides of the head. The presence of a sleep disturbance will usually define the underlying cause—difficulty falling asleep due to anxiety, and early or frequent awakening to depression. Chronic tension-type headaches usually are seen in women between ages thirty and fifty.

If the tension-type headaches occur intermittently (two or three times per month), and are controlled by over-the-counter (OTC) analgesics, the need to see a physician is not important. However, if the headaches occur several times per week, or are prolonged over several days, consultation with a physician is indicated. With these frequent headaches, and continuous use of OTC pain relievers, a phenomenon known as "rebound" may occur. Rebound is best described as an increasing need for a medication (OTC or prescription), and skipping or missing a dose will result in a headache. The individual will then take a dose of the suspect drug, and may require a higher dose—and continues the cycle. School or work conflicts, or marital and family relationships, are commonly linked to chronic tension-type headaches. You may want to examine your methods of coping with stress with your physician.

Treatment for chronic tension-type headaches is based on the source of the condition. If the headaches are due to anxiety (patient has difficulty falling asleep), treatment usually consists of a mild anxiolytic (antianxiety) drug. However, if the headaches are due to depression (patient experiences frequent or early awakening), the treatment primarily consists of antidepressants (discussed in chapter 10), biofeedback (discussed in chapter 8), and counseling.

Organic headaches are those headaches due to a physical disorder, such as a brain tumor or blood clot, and can be life-threatening. These headaches require immediate attention—a consult with a specialist and possibly, depending on the cause, neurosurgical intervention.

Vascular headaches (cluster and migraine) gain their name from the process by which the blood vessels of the brain expand or dilate, and cause the pain of cluster or migraine attacks.

Cluster headaches are typified by the brief duration of the acute attacks, lasting from fifteen minutes to three hours and occurring from once every other day to eight times a day. The pain is always unilateral, remaining on one side of the head during the entire series. Many cluster patients will complain of localized pain around or behind one eye. The pain has been described as stabbing, boring, or sharp knifelike sensations in the eye, and of such severity that patients have contemplated suicide during a cluster series. These headaches have also been called ciliary or migrainous neuralgia, histaminic cephalalgia, vidian and Sluder's neuralgia, and Horton's headache.

The defining characteristic of cluster headaches is the occurrence in a series—ranging from a few weeks to three or four months. This condition has been labeled cluster headache because of its occurrence in cycles or series. During a series, the headache may occur several times per day, usually waking the patient at the same time each night. In contrast to the patient experiencing an acute migraine attack, who will recline in a dark, quiet room, the patient enduring a cluster episode prefers to be upright and walking about the room. Associated symptoms include involuntary tearing, nasal congestion or runny nose, facial flushing, and swelling of the eyelid on the same side of the headache.

These headaches are more frequent in the spring and fall. Ninety percent of cluster headache sufferers are male and will note the first occurrence of these headaches during their twenties or thirties. The cluster series is self-limiting, usually continuing for a few weeks to several months. For some unfortunate individuals, the cluster headaches do not abate, and the individual will not experience a remission of these headaches for intervals lasting longer than fourteen days. This condition, chronic cluster headaches, is difficult to manage.

Up until a few years ago, the cause of cluster headache was unknown. A famous cluster headache researcher, Karl Ekbom of Sweden, treated a patient who suffered from both cluster headache and manic-depressive psychosis. Ekbom treated this patient, over a six-month period, for the manic phase with lithium. In addition to helping the patient's mania, during that interval, the patient's cluster headaches also subsided. Further use of lithium for cluster headaches has been successful and has led us to deduce that the hypothalamus (a part of the brain lying adjacent to the pituitary gland, which also controls emotions) is responsible for both manic-depressive psychosis and cluster headaches. Recent PET scanning (a special form of imaging), performed during an acute cluster attack, has further substantiated this theory. Also, a recent report in the journal *Neurology* described a patient experiencing the associated symptoms of a cluster headache (nasal congestion, swelling of the eyelid, etc.) without suffering from a headache.

Although the provocateur for a cluster series is unknown, during a series alcohol is a well-recognized trigger of the acute attacks. Researchers have precipitated a cluster attack using nitroglycerin tablets sublingually (placed under the tongue), or histamine injected subcutaneously (just under the skin). Cluster headache patients should also decrease or stop smoking during a series, as the intensity and duration of the acute attacks appear to be affected by this habit.

It would be impossible to improve on the following description by Frank Capra, the great film director, of an acute cluster headache attack. At age sixty-three, without warning, Capra suffered his first cluster headache. In *The Name Above the Title*, he writes:

We were caroling the birth of 1961 in the La Quinta Hotel dining room, when suddenly—a huge phantom bird sank three talons of its angry claw deep into my head and face, and tried to lift me. No warnings, nor preliminary signs. Just wham! A massive, killing pain over my right eye.

I clutched my head, stumbled out to the broad lawns, and skulked along oleander hedges to the deserted tennis courts. And there in the darkness, I moaned, panted, ballooned my cheeks, blew out short bursts of air, licked hot lips, wiped tears that poured out of my right eye, and clawed at my head, trying to uproot the fiendish talons from their iron grip.

One racking hour later, the talons let go. The paroxysm eased as suddenly as it had convulsed. Euphoria set in.

Episodic cluster headaches usually are treated with methysergide (discussed in chapter 10). Although long-term use of methysergide is associated with serious side effects, such as fibrous disorders of the heart, lung, and kidney, this drug's use in cluster headache treatment is usually brief. Corticosteroids, which are known as anti-inflammatory agents, are also used for episodic cluster headache treatment. Again, long-term use is not recommended, but the brief duration of cluster series does not prevent the use of the corticosteroids. Lithium is the treatment of choice for chronic cluster headaches.

The focus of this book will be on the other type of vascular headache—migraine. We will look at its mechanisms, variations, diagnosis, and treatment.

The term "migraine" comes from the French and is derived from the Greek word *hemicrania,* which means "half a head." The earliest recorded description of headache was included on the Ebers papyrus, which dates to Mesopotamia in 4000 B.C. when Tiu, the evil spirit of headache, supposedly attacked a victim:

> *Headache roameth over the desert, blowing like the wind.*
> *Flashing like lightning, it is loosed above and below.*
> *It cutteth off like a reed him who feareth not his god*
> *Like a stalk of henna, it slitteth his thews.*
> *It wasteth the flesh of him who hath no protecting goddess.*
> *Flashing like a heavenly star, it commeth like the dew;*
> *It standeth hostile against the wayfarer, scorching him like*
>   *the day.*
> *This man it hath struck and*
> *Like one with heart disease he staggereth.*
> *Like one bereft of reason he is broken.*

The Mechanism of Migraine

At one time, scientists believed that migraine was caused exclusively by abnormal swelling or dilation of the blood vessels entering the brain and the blood vessels in the covering of the brain (dura mater, pia mater). Many of the remarkable discoveries of medications that cut short a migraine attack or eliminated the attacks at their earliest onset were based on the drugs' effects on the blood vessels and receptors or nerve terminals that control these blood vessels. However, many newer imaging devices that now allow migraine researchers to observe the patient's brain during a migraine attack have led to a new theory about the mechanism of migraine.

Researchers are now able to show that during a migraine attack, there are more abnormally excitable neurons (the nerve cells) in the brain. Using a magnetoencephalogram—an instrument that is used to locate the magnetic source in the brain responsible for the magnetic fields—a group of scientists in Copenhagen (Jes Olesen, Martin Lauritzen) have shown that in certain migraine attacks that have been deliberately triggered, there is a spread of nervous activity that goes across the top of the brain and back down to the brain stem, where the vital pain centers are located. It has been shown that this spreading electrical activity is located in the brain stem of patients suffering from migraine but not from other types of headache. Researchers believe that the pain of migraine arises either from the activation from the brain stem pain centers or the blood vessels surrounding the brain. During a migraine attack, these blood vessels are stimulated to swell or dilate, or get a secondary inflammation due to a nerve located in the area known as the fifth cranial (trigeminal) nerve. This process is known as the trigeminal vascular reflex.

This finding is important because it will lead to more research that may tell us, down the road, how certain medications that control the excitable brain cells (mainly the anticonvulsants) selectively may be helpful in the prevention of migraine attacks. It is important to know that it takes various triggers to start this electrical sequence. The triggers may be diet, stress, or variations in hormone levels (i.e., menstrual periods).

In 1926, a substance that we continue to use today—ergotamine—for migraine treatment was identified. Ergotamine can either curtail a migraine attack or prevent the attack from starting. The results with ergotamine led to the further research of Harold G. Wolff.

In his pioneering work during the 1930s, Wolff identified four dynamic events occurring in a migraine attack:

1. The warning stage (aura)
2. Extracranial (outside the brain) vasodilation (swelling of the blood vessels), which may be the cause of migraine pain
3. Sterile inflammation, which increases pain and prolongs the acute migraine attack
4. Secondary muscle contraction

Wolff showed that the warning phase or aura of migraine was first produced by a constriction (narrowing) or a lack of oxygen to the blood vessels of the brain. He also showed that the pain of migraine was caused by a swelling or vasodilation of the blood vessels. In addition, there was a chemical pain-threshold-lowering substance involved in migraine—a process Wolff termed "sterile inflammation." Wolff described migraine as a self-limited neurogenic, sterile inflammation. He believed that the vasoconstriction (narrowing of the blood vessels) occurring during the aura usually had concluded before the extracranial vasodilation began.

After Wolff's research, researchers measuring blood flow during a migraine substantiated the theory of vascular changes occurring in the migraine evolution. An Italian pharmacologist and headache researcher, Federigo Sicuteri, established that during a migraine attack, there were changes in the blood-protein-like hormone serotonin. Sicuteri demonstrated that the blood serotonin increased before a headache and the blood vessels constricted—giving credence to Wolff and his idea of the causation of the migraine aura. He also showed that serotonin levels were markedly decreased during a headache and that during the pain phase of the attack, serotonin and its products were given off in large amounts in the urine of a migraineur. It was shown by other researchers that platelets, the primary blood substances that contain serotonin, group together and break up just prior to a migraine attack. Also, substances like serotonin that affect the blood vessels have been implicated and shown to be altered during migraine attacks. These substances include noradrenaline, the neurokinins, and the prostaglandins.

During the 1980s, Martin Lauritzen and Jes Olesen published findings that questioned the theories of Wolff. These investigators injected xenon-133, a radioactive isotope, into the carotid artery of migraine sufferers. They then induced a migraine attack, and performed arteriography—a method to visualize the blood vessels by injecting a dye or by inserting a catheter into a blood vessel. After this particular test, the researchers observed what they described as a wave of decreased impulses, slowly passing from the front of the brain to its back. They called it a "spreading oligemia"—a deficiency of blood in the body, an organ, or tissue. The oligemia continued after the essential migraine symptoms abated. These investigators concluded that the painless aura phase of migraine was possibly secondary to the spreading depression originally described by the Brazilian neurophysiologist A. A. P. Leão, and was not due to the oligemia. The spreading depression is a lack of electrical activity in the brain. In an earlier study, Olesen had noted that the oligemia did not occur in migraine without aura.

The results of these investigations have been disputed. Thomas Skyhøj Olsen's group (also from Copenhagen) have proposed that the "spreading oligemia" observed in cerebral (brain) fluid (CBF) studies during an acute migraine with aura may indicate a gradual decrease of cerebral fluid in an area that does not change size. The findings of this second group of researchers support the theory that migraine with aura and migraine without aura are due to the same disease process, and are not distinct. However, these two forms of migraine do vary in their degree of vasospasm (abnormal contraction of a blood vessel) and reduction of cerebral fluid.

More recently, a German research group utilized PET scanning in their investigations. PET scanning is a scan using radioactive material to measure and visualize the activity of an organ such as the brain (as opposed to an MRI or CT scan, which views the anatomy or structure of the organ). The German investigators suggested that the brain stem is the source of migraine.

The Acute Migraine Headache

During the attack, the severe throbbing is caused by the expansion or dilation of the blood vessels of the brain. Characteristically, the pain of migraine is limited to one side of the head and remains one-sided throughout the attack. However, the pain may radiate to the other side. Some migraine sufferers complain of pain on both sides of the head or across the forehead but claim that the pain is more severe on one side.

It bears repeating that migraine does not occur on a daily basis. The sufferer may experience an acute migraine attack every one to two months, or the headache may occur as often as two or three times weekly. The pain may last only a few hours, or it may continue for an entire day. Occasionally, the attack is prolonged and lasts two or three days—this is known as status migraine. These prolonged attacks are believed to be due to an inflammation (swelling) that surrounds the dilated blood vessel. Until that inflammation disappears, the blood vessel will remain widened, and the headache and its associated symptoms will continue.

Nausea, vomiting, and sensitivity to light (photophobia) are the most common associated symptoms of migraine. Some migraine sufferers report relief of their head pain after vomiting. If the vomiting with an acute attack is severe, dehydration may occur and the patient will require fluid replacement that may necessitate hospital admission.

During a migraine attack, the headache victim usually will seek relief by lying down in a darkened room. The migraine sufferer may complain of disturbances in hearing and balance during a headache. Many patients complain of phonophobia—that is, loud noises greatly disturb them during a headache. Patients also may complain of distorted hearing, finding their own or someone else's voice unreal and unnatural.

The headache also may be associated with sensitivity to odors, fatigue, dizziness or light-headedness, weakness in an arm or leg, ringing in the ears, tearing of either eye, nasal congestion or postnasal drip, facial flushing, sweating, or difficulty with vision. In the headache and preheadache stages, some patients note that they do not urinate as much or as frequently. As the headache decreases, they urinate an increased amount.

Slight mental changes may occur during an attack, including restlessness, confusion of ideas, and depression. A transient memory loss may also occur. These mental changes may be the first symptoms of the headache attack or they may follow the visual warning symptoms. These mental changes will rarely last longer than fifteen to twenty minutes. Before an attack, a patient may occasionally feel elated and full of energy.

The most persistent and distressing symptom of the migraine attack is the headache, but these sensory or mental symptoms are the most alarming, especially for patients experiencing them for the first time. The sensory symptoms are also very frightening if they continue for a long time or have a sudden onset for the first time in adult life. Usually by adulthood, the migraine attacks have established a predictable pattern and the patient knows what to expect during a headache attack.

The degree of pain varies from mild to severe, and the headache's pattern usually does not change throughout the patient's headache history. During the acute attack, the pain begins gradually and slowly increases in intensity. The pain may subside very slowly or disappear very quickly. The duration of the migraine pain varies from a few hours to one day, and up to three days, although abortive medications can affect the duration. At the beginning of the acute attack, the pain may be very severe and continue through-

33

out the attack, or it may decrease in intensity as the attack subsides. The headache rarely wakes the patient but will be present when the individual awakens.

Although the headache begins on one side, the pain becomes generalized in about one-third of the cases. When pain localizes to one site, it most often occurs in the temple. The area where the pain is confined can almost be outlined by the index finger. The pain may also start in the eyeball, the back of the neck, or a small spot on the forehead. It is often described as a boring sensation—as if an instrument were being forced into the skull. Eventually, the pain radiates over one side or to the rest of the head. If the pain starts at the back of the head, it may radiate over the head to the forehead or it may travel from one side or the back of the head to the neck or possibly into the arm. The pain may switch sides during a headache and end on the same side on which it started. Local tenderness does not usually occur during the migraine attack except over the "superficial temporal artery" (the prominent artery below the hairline on the side of the forehead).

If the pain is one-sided and can be felt over a large area, it is usually on the side opposite to that affected by the aura. In migraine with aura, the pain usually starts when the aura is declining and lasts several hours, sometimes for the remainder of the day.

What Is Migraine?

Migraine Triggers

Many factors can trigger an acute migraine attack, and stress is a major precipitating factor. Examples of stress include studying for exams, loss of a job, marital problems, or a death in the family. Quite often, the migraine sufferer is headache-free during a crisis but becomes incapacitated by a severe headache when the crisis has resolved. Some migraine patients internalize their emotions and these repressed feelings will trigger an acute attack.

Fatigue can also be a precipitant of migraine. It is important for the migraine sufferer to establish normal sleep patterns to prevent the acute attacks. Migraine headaches often occur when a patient is overtired. However, oversleeping can also bring on an acute attack. Many sufferers who complain of a "weekend" or "holiday" headache sleep late on their days off and fail to eat breakfast or drink their morning coffee at the regular time. Upon awakening, they complain of a severe headache that may continue throughout the day. This headache may be prevented if they set their alarm at the regular waking hour, get up, drink or eat something—and then return to bed if they wish.

The role of diet in migraine has been controversial. Elimination diets have been helpful in 30 percent to 40 percent of migraine sufferers. Many headache experts advise their patients to avoid foods containing tyramine, an amino acid that dilates the blood vessels. Foods that contain tyramine or other vasoactive substances include aged cheese; smoked, pickled or fermented foods; most alco-

35

holic beverages, especially red wines; nuts; chocolates; and citrus fruits. Other foods to avoid are processed meats such as hot dogs, bacon, ham, and salami. When these meats are processed or cured, sodium nitrite is added, and nitrites tend to dilate the blood vessels. A recommended "headache diet" will be presented in chapter 7.

Monosodium glutamate (MSG), which is used extensively in Chinese cooking, can provide a generalized reaction, including a headache—the phenomenon is sometimes known as the "Chinese restaurant syndrome." In some people, MSG can trigger a migraine headache.

Excessive amounts of caffeine can set off a headache and the migraine sufferer's intake of caffeine-containing beverages should be limited. These beverages include coffee, tea, hot chocolate, and many carbonated beverages. Limits should also be placed on over-the-counter analgesics that contain caffeine. Researchers at Loma Linda University have cited fat in foods as a migraine trigger and state that a reduction in fat may help or cure migraine. However, the studies on which this theory is based are not appropriately structured to make this theory convincing.

Dieting or fasting may provoke an acute migraine attack. If a person complains of headache after missing a meal, it does not necessarily mean that the sufferer has hypoglycemia or low blood sugar. Rather, it may indicate that he or she suffers from migraine. A decrease in the sugar content of the blood causes expansion of the blood vessels in the brain. For migraine sufferers, it is vital to maintain regularity in their daily living patterns in order to avoid headaches. The patient should eat three well-balanced meals daily at set times and avoid oversleeping. Dieting can cause the individual to skip a meal and will alter the body's normal blood sugar level, which may bring on a headache.

Excessive cigarette smoking can aggravate migraines and other types of vascular headaches. Migraine sufferers should discontinue smoking, or at least decrease their intake to ten cigarettes daily. Certain odors, such as cigar smoke, may also provoke a migraine.

Other factors may trigger a migraine, such as weather, barometric pressure, or altitude changes. The migraine sufferer must learn to identify the factors that influence the attacks in order to avoid them. However, avoidance of the provoking mechanism may not be the complete solution in preventing migraine attacks. Attacks will occur in spite of all precautions.

The Warning Phase

The symptoms of the aura usually affect vision, and include:

- Flashing lights
- Zigzag or jagged lines

- Blind spots
- Difficulty in focusing
- Distorted perception

The auras may be manifested by distorted figures—images out of focus or figures whose size is disproportionate—and are often referred to as the "Alice in Wonderland" syndrome.

Another occasional warning symptom is difficulty in speech, such as difficulty in finding the right word or using wrong words in speaking or writing. A complete inability to speak occurs on very rare occasions. Word deafness, the inability to understand what has been said may occur. The headache may also be preceded by "motor aphasia," the inability to say what the speaker wants to say. In right-handed migraine sufferers, difficulty in speech may accompany visual disturbances in the right eye as well as pins-and-needles sensations on the right side of the body. The reverse is true for left-handed sufferers.

Other warning signs can include any or all of the following:

- Tingling of the lips, face, or hands
- Weakness in an arm or leg
- Slight speech abnormality
- Watery eyes
- Loss of appetite
- Nasal congestion
- Sweating

- Confusion
- Restlessness

Some migraine sufferers may notice a terrible odor about their own body shortly before the headache. It is difficult to convince these people that the odor is not actually present.

Eighty percent of migraine sufferers have migraine without aura with the headache starting spontaneously and without warning. However, some individuals note a premonition that the headache is starting from twelve to thirty-six hours before the actual headache. The symptoms are vague, beginning imperceptibly, and develop slowly. The premonitory symptoms vary and may contrast, such as:

- Euphoria (feeling high) or becoming withdrawn
- Hyperactive or sluggish and clumsy
- Craving for food or anorexia
- Diarrhea or constipation
- Increased or frequent urination versus fluid retention

Other symptoms include:

- Yawning and fatigue
- Difficulty focusing
- Changes in personality
- Slurred speech
- Impaired concentration

- Irritability
- Agitation
- Sensitivity to light or sound
- Stiff neck
- General muscle weakness
- Sensitive skin
- Thirst

The patient may have a feeling of well-being, talkativeness, and a surge of energy. The famous neurologist Charles Airing was a migraine sufferer who had these episodes of excess energy prior to a migraine attack. In the few days prior to a migraine, he was able to write two scientific papers. This was a consistent pattern with his migraine attacks—and a very productive one.

Family and friends may notice that, prior to the headache, the individual face is pale, and the eyes appear dark, heavy, or sunken. The migraine victim may not be conscious of these warning symptoms, but a relative or friend may notice them.

The case study by Thomas Willis of Lady Conway in the sixteenth century is one of the most illustrative of the various premonitory symptoms before a headache.

. . . beautiful and young woman, indued with a slender habit of body, and an hot blood, being obnoxious to an hereditary headach, was wont to be afflicted with frequent and wandering fits of it, to wit, some upon every light occasion, and some of their own accord;

that is arising, without any evident cause. On the day before the coming of the spontaneous fit of this disease, growing very hungry in the evening, she eat a most plentiful supper, with an hungry, I may say a greedy appetite; presaging by this sign, that the pain of the head would most certainly follow the next morning; and the event never faled this augury. For as soon as she awaked, being afflicted by a most sharp torment, thorow the whole forepart of her head, she was troubled also with vomiting, sometimes of an acid, and as it were a bitriolock, humor, and sometimes of a cholerick and highly bitterish; hence according to this sign this headach is thought to arise from the vice of the stomach.

Case Report

Mike Hudson was a forty-one-year-old college professor who was divorced. He came to the clinic with the complaint of only one type of headache—a hard, sick headache that he had been experiencing since starting a new medication for arthritis. Mike remembered headaches occurring in childhood, at about age eleven. By the time he started high school, the headaches had all but disappeared, with rare attacks during college and graduate school. However, the headaches restarted in earnest about one year ago.

Mike was complaining of about two to three headaches per month, which last twelve to twenty-four hours. Sleep usually resolved the headache, and on occasion, he felt better after vomiting. He described the headaches as moderate to severe, but never incapacitating. The headaches were always one-sided, over the eye and ear. During childhood, the headaches were on both sides, but these current headaches are never bilateral. He noted that the headaches were of pounding quality with some neck soreness.

Although Mike did not experience an aura, he was extremely irritable and anxious starting about two days before headache onset. The headaches were associated with nausea, occasional vomiting, sensitivity to light and sound, and blurred vision. He did try to work with a headache, but it could be difficult to write or do any research. He tried elimination diets but did not identify any food trigger. He did get headaches on weekends if he slept too long. Mike had not linked the headaches to any weather changes. For the acute headache, he used aspirin or ibuprofen. After he started having chronic pain in his knees, his family physician started him on indomethacin for osteoarthritis—he recalled that he started that medication about one month prior to this recent onset of headaches. I believed that Mike was suffering from migraine without aura, which was probably induced by the indomethacin (Indocin). After consulting with Mike's family physician, I discontinued the indomethacin and started Mike on another nonsteroidal anti-inflammatory, ketoprofen (commonly known as Orudis). The headaches decreased after six weeks on this regimen, and he noted that the knee pain was somewhat relieved.

Headache Resolution

How does a migraine attack end? If drugs are not used, will the headache just disappear? Yes, but it may take several days—and the patient will endure unnecessary pain and disability due to the migraine attack. When the headache resolves, the migraine victim may notice another set of symptoms. These symptoms can last from one hour to four days, and on average twenty-three hours.

Often, at the end of the attack, some individuals feel "drained," while others may feel "better than normal." The following have been noted as "postdromal" symptoms, occurring after the attack: euphoria, feeling blue, slow intellect, impaired concentration, irritability, lifelessness, muddled state, inattentiveness or sluggishness, aching muscles, and excessive yawning. Although the migraine victim may feel like returning to work, his or her creativity and mental acuity may be diminished. Following the attack, the migraine victim may have little appetite and may favor a meal that is light, such as tea and toast, or a soft-boiled egg. Others have noted an increased desire for sweets—even a craving for chocolate. Some may have increased urination and thirst, while others will have decreased urine output. Many migraine sufferers will describe the end of the headache as similar to a "hangover." The headache may even reoccur—briefly—if they shake their head or bend down.

It is possible that some of these postheadache symptoms are, in reality, the aftereffects of the drugs that have been used to stop or relieve the headache. However, these symptoms have been reported in individuals who have not used drug therapy. These migraine sufferers may have used self-help methods, including sleep, to relieve the pain of the migraine attack.

But how do we recognize the types of headache, and establish a diagnosis? In my own experience, I have developed certain observation techniques with headache patients:

- A person with migraine with aura is often (but not always) high-strung, likes to talk in rather quick and hurried phrases, and is extraordinarily neat and well groomed—a type-A personality who can be a nitpicker and is precise. This person will describe himself or herself as a perfectionist. When I return to the examining room, after the patient has dressed after the physical exam, the patient will have carefully folded the paper gown and lined up the chair so it is even with the wall or table.

- A person with a headache due to anxiety or depression is likely to appear quite calm and relaxed, although he or she is complaining of severe, disabling headaches.

- An individual who does not swing his or her arms while walking may have a headache due to an organic problem of the brain or the central nervous system.

- A person who makes every effort to avoid certain spots on the face, such as not putting makeup on one part of the cheek or not shaving one area of the face, may have a pain disorder associated with trigger points—trigeminal neuralgia.

- A person who has trouble talking or articulating words, and who is right-handed, may have a lesion on the left side of the brain. The speech center in the brain on a right-handed person is on the left side of the brain. When a speech difficulty occurs in the presence of a headache, it suggests that a serious disease, such as a brain tumor or aneurysm, is present.

- During the examination, I look at the patient's skin to get a clue about his or her headache problem. Cluster headache patients often have thick facial skin, with deep furrows in the forehead, and pitted, coarse skin on the cheeks—something like the skin on an orange.

Diagnosing Migraine

How will you know that you are experiencing a migraine? Let's review the "clinical picture" of a migraine through a typical headache history. The questions below should help you recognize if your headaches are migraine. It is important that your diagnosis be confirmed by a physician. Your headache history and physical examination will help the physician rule out any organic or serious causes of the headache. This list of questions is repeated in the back of the book with space for your own answers. There are no objective tests for migraine. However, the physician may order laboratory tests and neuroradiologic examinations (CT scan or MR imaging) to make certain that you do not have a serious underlying cause of your headaches. The testing may also help the physician determine what type of treatment is appropriate for you.

• *How many types of headache do you experience?*

It is important for the physician to know if you are experiencing more than one type of headache: Do you have a daily mild-to-moderate headache as well as a more severe, less frequent headache? The presence of more than one type of headache will impact on the diagnosis as well as the treatment selected for you. Coexisting migraine and tension-type headache will be discussed in chapter 4.

• *How long have you suffered from headaches? At what age did your headaches start?*

One key to a diagnosis of migraine is the age at which the attacks start. Typically, migraine headaches start during adolescence or the twenties. However, migraine can begin in childhood. Migraine rarely begins after age forty, but it is possible for the headaches to start later in life. If the initial or first headache starts after the age of fifty, the patient should have a thorough physical and neurological workup to rule out a physical cause for the headache. Quite often migraines decrease or disappear as a person ages.

- *How often do the headaches occur?*

For most migraine sufferers, the headache will occur one to eight times per month. Many female migraineurs will relate the headache to their monthly period. Other migraine sufferers may go several months without a headache. It is important to remember that migraine is not a "daily headache." In 1981, with Dr. José Medina, I identified a rare form of migraine, known as "cyclic migraine." This type is characterized by its frequent occurrence—twelve times per month. It is usually responsive to lithium therapy, similar to the treatment for chronic cluster headaches discussed earlier.

- *Where is the pain located?*

Migraine headache is typically one-sided, although it can affect both sides of the head, or change sides during a headache. The pain may be located at the temples or at the back of the head.

- *How long does a headache last?*

Migraine usually lasts from eight to twenty-four hours. However, prolonged migraine attacks that last over twenty-four hours are termed "status migraine."

- *How severe is the headache?*

Migraine pain is usually severe and can be incapacitating. Often, the patient is disabled from several hours to several days because of the pain and its associated symptoms.

- *How would you describe the pain?*

Migraine headaches are frequently described as throbbing or pulsating, and physical exertion may increase the severity.

- *Do you have any warning symptoms of an impending headache?*

The presence of a set of warning symptoms divides migraine into two types—migraine with aura (classic migraine) and migraine without aura (common migraine). The aura or warning stage is evident in about 20 percent of migraine sufferers. These warning signs can occur thirty to sixty minutes before the onset of a migraine headache. Usually, the aura involves visual symptoms, such as loss of part of your visual field, seeing bright stars or jagged lines, or experiencing blind spots. Some patients will describe visual hallucinations, such as those depicted by Lewis Carroll in *Through the Looking Glass*. The famed abbess, Hildegard of Bingen, created beautiful tapestries that are attributed to the symptoms of a migraine aura. Other symptoms may be included in the migraine aura, such as numbness in an arm, leg, or both. The aura does not have to precede each migraine attack. As migraine sufferers age, they may experience the aura without a headache following it.

There are other symptoms that may be associated with migraine with aura, as in the following case.

Case Report

Frannie Dougherty was a thirty-five-year-old nurse with a long history of headaches. She only reports one type of headache, which originally started while she was a teenager. As she recalled, the headaches started about the same time as her menstrual periods. She was now experiencing one to two headaches per month, with one usually occurring at menses. The headaches lasted about eight to sixteen hours if she did not take any medication. The headaches were very severe, and could be incapacitating—she had ten sick days last year, all because of a headache. The headaches were always one-sided, on either side, usually above the eye, and would sometimes radiate to the back of the head. She described the headache as throbbing and pulsating.

Frannie had been experiencing aura symptoms since the original headaches started. The aura began about thirty minutes prior to the onset of headache, and she saw bright, zigzag lines, and occasionally blind spots. However, the aura did not always precede the headache. Frannie was especially bothered with the associated symptoms of the attack—extreme nausea and vomiting, sensitivity to light, light-headedness, and skin pallor. During the past three years, she was admitted to the community hospital because she became dehydrated from the excessive vomiting. She noted that the headaches were precipitated by chocolate and red wine, as well as her menses. Also, she experienced a migraine after almost every plane trip. When she

first married, she started taking birth control pills, and that was when she noticed an increase in her headaches. During her two pregnancies, the headaches disappeared after the fourth month, and they were mild while she was breast-feeding her daughters. Because of the increase in headaches related to the birth control pills, she opted for surgical sterilization and underwent a tubal ligation (tying her fallopian tubes). However, the headaches continued to occur at menses despite being off the Pill.

When Frannie experienced a headache, her choice of treatment was limited. The vomiting could continue for over twenty-four hours, and it started almost as soon as the headache started. The fact that the primary associated symptoms of migraine are nausea and vomiting, and a sluggishness of the gastrointestinal system (stomach and intestines), precluded the use of drugs taken by mouth.

She was delighted when sumatriptan (Imitrex) injections were introduced, and she now uses the sumatriptan nasal spray (see chapter 9). Frannie felt that she should start preventive therapy (chapter 10) so that she wouldn't miss work and she could get on with her life. I told Frannie that her headaches were migraine with aura, and we certainly could initiate prophylactic therapy. (The choices for preventive therapy are numerous and are further described in chapter 10.)

Some migraine patients—those with or without aura—may sense an impending attack with vague symptoms. They may feel extremely hungry or tired before a headache, or they may lose their appetite or have a burst of energy prior to a severe headache. These "premonitory" symptoms of migraine may occur twelve to thirty-six hours before the start of an actual migraine.

• *Are any other symptoms associated with your headaches?*

Migraine is known as a "sick headache," since it may be accompanied by nausea, vomiting, and extreme sensitivity to light. Other associated symptoms include dizziness, blurred vision, sensitivity to sound, and irritability. The disabling nature of a migraine attack is related to both the pain of the headache as well as these other complaints. Treatment is especially complicated by the associated symptoms of nausea and vomiting, as demonstrated by Frannie's case.

• *Do you have a sleep disturbance?*

Migraine patients will relate that the headache is present upon awakening. However, for patients experiencing coexisting migraine and tension-type headaches, difficulty falling asleep or frequent and early awakening may be a prominent feature of the patient's condition.

• *Is there a family history of headache?*

Most experts believe that migraine is a hereditary disease, as about 70 percent of migraine sufferers have a family history of migraine. Recently, researchers have identified a chromosome—chromosome 19—that they believe is a genetic link to migraine. The incidence of migraine is especially high if both parents have suffered from migraine.

- *Are the headaches related to the menstrual cycle?*

Seventy percent of migraine sufferers are female, and 70 percent of those women will relate a link between their headaches and their periods. The initial onset of migraine may be associated with the start of their periods. They may experience a migraine at the time of ovulation, or immediately before, during, or after the period. Typically, the migraine patient will report that their headaches disappear after the third month of pregnancy. Postmenopausal migraine sufferers may notice a gradual decrease and then disappearance of the migraine attacks. Estrogen used in hormonal supplements and birth control pills is known to increase the frequency, severity, duration, and complications of migraine. These issues will be explored in the next chapter.

- *Is there a seasonal relationship to the headaches?*

Migraine attacks are often related to changes in weather or barometric pressure. The headaches may increase with changes in altitude—such as a vacation in the mountains. Also, the stress associated with the holidays may precipitate a migraine attack. I do see an increase in migraine attacks during spring and autumn.

- *Are there any specific triggers to your headache?*

Certain food items may be related to the headache and they are described in chapter 7. Migraine patients are especially sensitive to foods containing the amino acid tyramine (found in aged cheese, pickled or marinated foods, or yogurt). Chocolate, which contains the amino acid phenylethylamine, is a well-known migraine trigger. Alcoholic beverages are known to provoke migraine. Migraine patients may complain of a headache due to skipping or missing a meal; oversleeping on weekends or holidays; skipping a dose of caffeine, whether in a beverage or over-the-counter pain relievers; exertion, such as exercise, orgasm, and straining for a bowel movement (these headaches should be thoroughly investigated for serious organic causes); some medications:

1. Agents used for treating high blood pressure (minoxidil, reserpine)
2. Agents used for treating heart disease (nitrates)
3. Agents used for arthritis (indomethacin)
4. Estrogen used in birth control pills and hormonal replacement therapy

- *How would you describe your personality? Do you notice any emotional factors in the occurrence of your headaches? Would you relate your headaches to stress? Do you have any significant problems at work, at school, or with your marriage or children?*

The existence of a "migraine personality" has been highly disputed. Some researchers contend that the migraine sufferer is usually a perfectionist, ambitious, compulsive, and very orderly. Of course, there are exceptions to the rule, such as the very easygoing migraine sufferer or the highly competitive, intense person who has never com-

53

plained of a headache. Many migraine patients, at their physician visits, will bring long and detailed lists of the headaches, medications, treatments, and various tests they have undergone. Quite often, migraine sufferers will build an environment for themselves that is so complex they are unable to cope with it. These individuals may serve on a number of committees or attempt to work full-time and keep a full class schedule. It is difficult to determine whether the personality traits or the stress of the person's busy life caused the headaches. Stress, and sometimes relief of stress, may be related to the precipitation of an acute headache. During the history, the physician may question you about your relationships—work, school, marital, and family. These issues are particularly important if you are experiencing more than one type of headache or if your migraine attacks are increasing in frequency or severity.

• *Are you on any medications for your headaches?*
The types of medications that you have found effective in combating the migraine attacks may confirm your diagnosis. For example, if your headaches respond to an agent containing an ergotamine, then you probably are suffering from a vascular type of headache, such as migraine. It is also important to know how much medication is needed to relieve the headache pain.

• *Are you on any other medications?*
As stated earlier, migraine can be triggered by some medications. For example, you may have suffered migraine

headaches as a young adult, but the headaches disappeared with menopause. Suddenly, the headaches have returned. Coincidentally, your physician is now treating your hypertension with minoxidil or reserpine. Or you may require nitroglycerin for angina, and you notice an increase in your headaches. Indomethacin (Indocin) an agent used for arthritis and certain headache problems, can actually precipitate a headache in sensitive individuals.

Migraine in Children

Headache is a common complaint in both children and adolescents. For many migraine sufferers, their initial headache occurs during childhood or while they are teenagers. In 69 percent of children with migraine, there is a family history of similar headaches.

The clinical features of migraine in children are:

- Recurrent headaches
- Relief after sleep
- Nausea, vomiting, and abdominal pain
- Throbbing or pounding quality of the headache
- One-sided headache

Prior to puberty, migraine is more prevalent in males. During adolescence, the pendulum swings to the females—who may relate the onset of their migraine attacks with menarche (the onset of menstrual periods). Children may experience migraine with, or without, aura. The premonitory symptoms are similar to those reported by adults, such as pallor, malaise, fatigue, and irritability. During an acute migraine attack, the child will often go to his or her bedroom, complaining of extreme sensitivity to light and sound. The child will often express a need to sleep, and the attack usually resolves within two to six hours.

Several triggers have been reported by children with migraine:

- Anxiety
- Minor head trauma
- Exercise
- Menses
- Travel
- Diet (chocolate, pizza, cola beverages)

It is important for the child and the parent to identify triggers, particularly food items. On occasion, elimination diets may be an easy intervention for childhood migraine.

Case Report

Kevin Strauss was a bright and active eleven-year-old boy. His headaches had started the year before, while he was in fifth grade. The headaches were moderate, and his mother related them to his dismay over sports and an especially strict teacher. Kevin wasn't growing as fast as some of his friends, and his inquisitiveness and socializing were not appreciated by his teacher. But by sixth grade, the headaches had increased—alarming his parents. Kevin underwent a physical and neurological examination—both normal. And, to assure his parents, I ordered a CT scan, which also was negative. I asked Kevin's mom to maintain a daily chart for the month—recording his headaches, and if possible marking any triggers. We asked Kevin's mom to have him follow an elimination diet—cutting out one food item at a time and then trying it again. If a headache occurred after the food item was reintroduced, it may be a factor in Kevin's headaches.

The Strausses returned six weeks later. They felt like detectives and were satisfied with their work—a pepperoni pizza, and one week later a chocolate milkshake, had preceded a migraine headache. But how do you keep an eleven-year-old boy away from pizza and chocolate? Kevin understood that these food items were contributing to his headaches, and was willing to cooperate. The headaches seemed to decrease for a while but then began to increase again. The Strausses were puzzled. We all—Kevin included—reviewed the headache chart. Kevin had given up his favorite chocolate milk drinks after school, but he was stopping at the local store and getting a caffeine beverage every day while walking home. After a discussion, we agreed that Kevin would switch to fruit juice or a noncaffeinated drink. The headaches decreased, and Kevin has actually celebrated a basketball victory with a pizza party (and no cola), and did not suffer a headache. It is possible that by the time Kevin is in high school, he can go back to a full diet with his favorites.

Treatment of childhood migraine is discussed in chapter 10. Selection of medications will be based on the patient's age, size, and frequency and severity of the headache. Biofeedback has shown excellent results in childhood migraine.

Establishing Your Own Headache History

In the Appendix of this book, you will find a headache calendar that is similar to the one given to Kevin and his parents. I would suggest maintaining this calendar for four to eight weeks and sharing the findings with your physician. Although you may not be suffering a daily headache, make an entry for each day—noting whether or not you experience a headache. Even if you don't get a headache, note on the calendar if you confronted a headache precipitant—stress, menses, food trigger. It may help you identify whether or not a common headache trigger really affects you.

If you do experience a headache, and use a drug for the headache—whether over-the-counter or prescribed—you should list the degree of relief that you obtained. You should also note the amount of the drugs that you consumed. This part of the chart will help your physician select appropriate therapy for you, and also help the doctor understand if you have developed a tolerance to a medication—that is, if you require more and more of a drug in order to obtain relief.

Also, we have included a list of the questions used in a headache history with space for your own answers. You may want to complete these questions and share the responses with your physician. This process will be especially helpful if you are consulting a headache specialist for the first time.

CHAPTER 2

Migraine and Women

Approximately 70 percent of migraine sufferers are female, and about 70 percent of those women relate the headaches to the menstrual cycle. Hormones play a pivotal role in these headaches. The various life stages of a woman will reflect the hormonal changes that occur and specific headache events at each phase—menstrual cycle, pregnancy, breast-feeding, perimenopausal, and postmenopausal.

In the origin of most headaches in women, hormones are probably involved. In this chapter, we will focus on migraine headaches as they relate to the hormones governing the menstrual cycle, pregnancy, menopause, and estrogen therapy (birth control pills and hormone replacement therapy). Because males also experience migraine, a link to the reproductive hormones does not fully explain the etiology of these conditions. However, it is the changing levels of these hormones, usually responding to some other physical signals, that are influential factors in triggering migraines in those genetically predisposed to these headaches.

Historical Perspectives

As early as 1666, Johannis Van der Linden, in *De Hemicrania Menstrua,* described menstrual headache as a one-sided headache associated with nausea and vomiting. The headache in question occurred monthly in proximity to the menstrual flow of Van der Linden's patient, the Marchioness of Brandenburg.

We are indebted to the work of Brian Somerville, who conducted the first careful analyses of the role of reproductive hormones in migraine. During the 1970s, Dr. Somerville recognized that migraine attacks usually occur just before or immediately after the onset of menstruation. He also noted that about five days before menstruation onset, estrogen and progesterone begin to drop from peak levels, falling to much lower levels immediately before menstrual bleeding. In his research, Somerville attempted to determine if the precipitating event of the migraine attack was due to the decline of estrogen or progesterone. Initially, he administered daily injections of progesterone to six women during the premenstrual phase—three to six days before the expected onset of menstruation. The injections continued until at least the second day of menstruation. Thus, the plasma level of progesterone was maintained in the usual premenstrual range, although estradiol levels declined normally. In four of six subjects, onset of menstruation was delayed. However, five of six experienced migraines at the usual time in their cycles.

Somerville also gave daily injections, premenstrually, of slow-release estrogen (estradiol) to eight women. For all patients, menstruation started on schedule; however, migraine attacks were delayed by three to nine days, at which time the levels of estrogen were again at preinjection levels. Seven patients experienced their usual attacks, albeit delayed, although the eighth subject reported no headache after the progesterone treatment and then experienced a less-severe migraine. In another trial, Somerville administered the estradiol injections to two women who were no longer menstruating—one menopausal and one who was failing to ovulate—and both had been migraine-free since cessation of menstruation. In these subjects, migraines developed after Somerville ceased estradiol injections and the women's estrogen levels declined. In reviewing the data, Somerville concluded that progesterone withdrawal causes menstrual bleeding but did not precipitate migraine. Estrogen withdrawal, in contrast, "plays a key role in the precipitation of menstrual migraine."

A variety of mechanisms for this effect were contemplated, including the action of estrogen either on blood vessels in the brain or on platelets, thus triggering the release of serotonin. Somerville later found that in order to provoke a migraine attack, he had to expose his subjects for several days to high estrogen levels and then decrease these levels. However, he was unsuccessful in his attempts to prevent migraine by premenstrual administration of oral estradiol or conjugated estrogen tablets (such as Premarin). These procedures also did not affect the normal decline in plasma estrogen.

Since Somerville's studies during the 1970s, menstrual headaches have been continually investigated. In later reviews, "menstrual migraine" was narrowly defined as acute migraine attacks that only occur two days before to three days after onset of menstruation.

Menstrual Migraine

True menstrual migraine as defined above is rare as opposed to menstrually associated attacks, which occur in 60 percent of patients. Patients with menstrually associated migraine attacks experience these headaches at menses, but can also suffer with migraine attacks at other times of the month. The origins of menstrual migraine are now considered to be caused by rapid fluctuations in the levels of estrogen and progesterone, in particular, or changes in the estrogen/progesterone ratio. It is these changes or variations in hormones that trigger the migraine attack as opposed to the stability of the hormones in men. The production of estrogen and progesterone by the ovaries is stimulated by both of these hormones, thus signaling the production of prostaglandins by the endometrium, which is the lining of the uterus.

Prostaglandins are fatty acids that act like hormones, and have good and bad functions. The bad functions can promote pain and headache. The good functions include their effects on the cardiovascular system, smooth muscle, and uterine contraction. If the prostaglandins are interrupted, the pain doesn't occur.

Dramatic shifts in estrogen levels have been reported to increase prostaglandin levels in women predisposed to migraine. Pain receptors are sensitized by prostaglandins, which also cause inflammation, resulting in pain. Levels of some prostaglandins increase during a migraine attack. Administering the prostaglandin E_1 into study subjects can produce the classic symptoms of migraine as well as abdominal cramping.

During migraine attacks, the release of the pituitary hormone prolactin may be enhanced by serotonin. Prolactin controls lactation (breast milk production). Elevated plasma levels of prolactin are produced by some of the major migraine precipitants, including stress, exercise, and oral contraceptives. Some migraine agents, such as the ergot alkaloids (chapter 9) and clonidine (chapter 10), also suppress prolactin production, confirming the theory that high prolactin levels are related to the development of migraine attacks and pain.

Sometimes, we see patients with prolactin-secreting tumors of the pituitary gland that are nonmalignant, and can cause migrainelike headaches. These tumors are

treated with a drug that acts as an antiprolactin agent—
bromocriptine. Bromocriptine, in most instances, will
shrink the tumor. Occasionally, surgical intervention is
needed.

Premenstrual Syndrome (PMS)

Headaches that occur during the premenstrual part of
women's menstrual cycles can be diagnosed as either tension-type headaches or a combination of migraine and
tension-type headaches. These patients may suffer with a
wide range of other PMS symptoms, both physical and
emotional. Physical complaints include fatigue, joint pain,
breast tenderness, fluid retention, and food cravings. The
individual may complain of emotional manifestations such
as anxiety, depression, impaired judgment or memory, and
paranoia. Fluctuations in estrogen and progesterone levels
are linked to both types of headaches.

Pregnancy

Migraine reportedly improves during pregnancy in about
70% of female migraineurs. This remission is linked to the
sustained high estrogen levels during pregnancy. If the migraine attacks continue during the first trimester (first 3

months of the pregnancy), the expectant migraine sufferer may note headache-free intervals during the last two trimesters. On the other hand, some individuals may experience an increase in either frequency or severity of the headaches during pregnancy. An initial onset of migraine during the first trimester has also been reported, due to the alterations of the hormones.

Postpartum

After delivery, during the postpartum period, the susceptible individual may again experience migraine attacks. Typically, these headaches will first occur from four to six days postpartum, although these headaches may occur at any time during the first week postpartum. If the headaches are of recent onset, a prior personal or family history of migraine will probably be reported.

The migraine attacks that occur during the postpartum period are related to the rapid decrease in estrogen and progesterone following delivery. The postpartum migraine attacks may be milder than previous attacks. Some women complaining of headaches during the postpartum period have reported more tension and depression. The headaches often coincided with weight loss, starting three or four days postpartum. Those headaches may be considered as part of the postpartum depression complex.

Menopause

As menopause approaches, estrogen levels and fluctuations gradually decrease—and migraines usually diminish in frequency or may resolve with menopause. In some patients, however, the migraine attacks can increase or an individual may experience the initial onset of migraine—particularly in women who are vulnerable to any changes in their hormone levels.

The cause of menopause, whether naturally occurring or surgically induced (via a hysterectomy), may have varying effects on headaches. In one study involving forty-seven postmenopausal migraine sufferers, the migraine attacks seemed to improve (67 percent) after physiological menopause but not after surgical menopause. This finding should preclude a female migraine sufferer from undergoing a hysterectomy to prevent her headaches. Migraine attacks that probably would have ceased ordinarily because of menopause can be increased by hormone replacement therapy (HRT), consisting of one or another form of estrogen and progesterone.

In patients receiving HRT, the increase in migraine attacks may manifest immediately after starting the therapy or have a gradual onset after prolonged usage. Recent-onset migraine or persistent headaches may actually be helped by continuous administration of HRT, in low daily dose treatments instead of cyclic treatment, which exposes the patient to higher doses for twenty-one days, followed by total removal of the estrogen for seven days. For my patients using HRT, I will consult with their family physician or gynecologist and recommend discontinuation of the hormone therapy. However, if the other physician or the patient insists on continuing the HRT, I recommend noncyclic therapy—and the use of the lowest possible doses of estrogen on a daily basis. If the patient was using cyclic estrogen, an acute migraine attack often occurred on those days when the patient was not taking the estrogen. It should be noted that whether the patient is receiving cyclic or noncyclic therapy, HRT can aggravate a migraine condition.

For several years, Dr. Edward Lichten has advocated the use of hormonal treatment for menstrually related migraines that do not respond to standard therapies. He reported in seventeen of twenty-four menopausal women that continuous oral or transdermal estrogen (skin patches) was beneficial in migraine therapy. His investigation also found that in menopausal women who reported a prior history of migraines, maintaining a specific serum estradiol level could prevent hormonally influenced migraines.

Case Report

Leah Antonacci was a fifty-one-year-old writer who was divorced and living with her son. She was suffering from one type of headache. The headaches originally started when she was twelve years old, and she recalled her menarche at eleven. At age forty-nine, because of excessive menstrual bleeding and dysmenorrhea (painful periods), Leah underwent a complete hysterectomy. Prior to her hysterectomy, she could experience three or four headaches per month, associated with mid month (ovulation) and her period.

Now, she was experiencing two headaches per month. The headaches varied in duration, from a few hours to two days. She noted that the headaches were one-sided, but encompassed one entire side of her head, and occasionally radiated to the other side of her head. The severity was moderate to incapacitating, and she had missed work on occasion due to the headaches. Leah described the headaches as a throbbing pain. She did not experience any aura symptoms or premonitory signs. The headaches were always associated with nausea, vomiting, sensitivity to light and odors, and difficulty concentrating. This made working during a headache very difficult.

After her hysterectomy, the gynecologist put Leah on cyclic hormone replacement therapy (HRT)—the estrogen supplement is to be taken for twenty-one days of each month followed by seven days off the medication. During the week she stops the medication, she experienced two headaches. During the last two trimesters of her pregnancy, she had been headache-free. Leah never noticed any link between her headaches and weather or altitude changes. Since she takes a skiing vacation every February, she would have remembered a headache ruining her vacation. I advised Leah that I felt she was suffering from migraine without aura, associated with HRT. In order to prevent these headaches, I recommended that Leah take continuous HRT, each day of the month. I also recommended that she use the estrogen replacement at the lowest possible dose.

In a particularly interesting report, a female migraine patient was given an estrogen skin patch. These drugs are replaced each week, and the patient has a continuous administration of estrogen. This patient did not report any increase in her headaches except when she attended an aerobic exercise class. It seems that when she was exercising, she sped up the absorption of the drug—she was, in fact, increasing her estrogen levels.

Oral Contraceptives and Headache

As could be expected, the use of oral contraceptives (birth control pills) can impact on those females who are prone to migraine. These agents may accentuate hormonal fluctuations, and thus can increase the frequency, duration, severity, and complications of migraine, particularly in those individuals with a prior history of migraine. Oral contraceptives may also induce initial onset of migraine. In such cases, a family history of migraine is usually present.

The most frequently reported side effect of oral contraceptive use is migraine headaches. More than one-fourth of the women in one study terminated the use of oral contraceptives because of headache. Over the past three decades, the pharmaceutical industry has continued to develop newer oral contraceptives with lower doses of estrogen, and the incidence of side effects, including headache, has decreased.

Case Report

Anika Sorensen was a member of a family of patients that I had managed for several years—in fact, she was third-generation. Her grandmother had been one of my earliest headache patients, and then I treated Anika's mother and two older sisters. Anika's mother, Ingrid, had asked me to see Anika when she was fourteen, and the onset of her migraine attacks coincided with her menarche. Anika had been involved in gymnastics since age nine, and her periods were delayed. After she stopped participating in gymnastics, Anika grew to be a willowy adolescent, with normal periods and the family "curse"—monthly migraine attacks. She initially responded well to the use of NSAIDs at period time (see chapter 10), and eventually stopped seeing me during her college years. Her mother proudly told me that Anika was managing her headaches and was doing quite well. She also told me that Anika seemed happier, that she had decided at Christmas to be straightforward with her parents and sisters—she had advised everyone that she was gay.

After college graduation, Anika pursued a career in politics, and was well known in her home state for her activities in the gay and lesbian community. While working on the political campaign of a congressional candidate, Anika's headaches had increased to more than once per month—she noted a real change in the headache pattern. She returned to the office, and because of this increase in her migraine attacks—in both severity and frequency—an MRI was ordered, and revealed no abnormality. I discussed all the possible reasons for an increase in headaches, including the stress of the upcoming election. I asked Anika to maintain a headache calendar so that we could identify some possible triggers.

Anika returned to the clinic two months later, accompanied by her older sister, Gretchen. They decided to incorporate their physician visit into a little shopping trip to the Chicago Loop. Although I don't normally see two patients at the same time, the two sisters opted to stay in the same examining room. When we reviewed Anika's headache chart, neither of us could identify a specific headache trigger. Suddenly, Gretchen slapped her hand on the desk, and said, as an older sister would, "Anika, I bet you never told Dr. Diamond that you went on the Pill. You know, the ones that are good for your complexion—they helped your acne." Anika blushed, and said, "You're right, I did forget to tell Dr. D., and my headaches started to increase about one month after I started those pills."

Considering Anika's lifestyle, I had never thought to ask her about using oral contraceptives. Anika had seen one of the TV commercials for Ortho Tri-Cyclen, which promote the fact that this particular birth control pill helps combat acne. After recovering from my shock, I advised Anika to discontinue the Pill, and we would see how the headaches were affected. Two months later, Anika phoned—the only headaches she had experienced during this interval were at period time. She was delighted with the decrease in headaches, and had consulted a dermatologist about her acne. I had also learned that I should never assume anything!

If Anika was primarily using the Pill for contraception, I would have recommended that she consider another form of birth control. If a patient does not want to stop the Pill, I recommend birth control pills with the lower doses of estrogen. I also prescribe the use of an NSAID during the week that the patient is not on an active drug. However, for individuals with migraine with aura, I am reluctant to continue the Pill, because these particular patients are more prone to complications, such as blood clots and stroke.

CHAPTER 3
Migraine in Relation to Other Diseases

Migraine has often been linked to other diseases, such as epilepsy and allergic disorders. Other vascular conditions—that is, disorders affecting the blood vessels—such as Raynaud's phenomenon, systemic lupus erythematosus, mitral valve prolapse, and multiple sclerosis, are reportedly associated with migraine. The presence of coexisting medical disorders (hypertension, arthritis, glaucoma) may impact on the choice of treatment options. Also, treatment for other medical conditions may exacerbate the headache problem. We will further discuss headache drug treatment in chapters 9 and 10.

Allergy

Many reports have linked migraine to allergic disorders, such as asthma, hay fever, hives, rhinitis, and eczema. Since both of these conditions are widespread, it is very likely that an individual will suffer from both disorders. There is no increased prevalence of allergic symptoms in migraine—in one study, 80 percent of migraine sufferers were actually free of any allergic disorder.

Allergy to foods has been considered as a migraine trigger. But as we discussed in the previous chapter, the vasoactive substance in certain foods (cheese, chocolate, red wine, hot dogs) can trigger a headache in susceptible individuals but are not necessarily allergies, and elimination diets are not the answer for every migraine sufferer.

Asthma

As with other allergic disorders, migraine has been linked to asthma—but it could be coincidental. The prevalence of asthma is increasing in the U.S. population, and it is probably that the migraine sufferer will also be suffering from asthma. For patients with aspirin-sensitive asthma, migraine treatment may pose an enormous challenge. These individuals are usually intolerant of the nonsteroidal anti-inflammatory drugs (NSAIDs), as well as the dyes used in some medications. For the migraine sufferer with concomitant asthma or other pulmonary problems, certain medications for migraine prevention cannot be used. For example, the beta blocker propranolol (commonly known as Inderal) is one of the most utilized preventive agents for migraine, but it cannot be used in asthmatic patients. The alternative agents that are safe for asthmatic patients are labeled "cardioselective" beta blockers—metoprolol and atenolol—and have been used successfully in migraine prophylactic therapy (chapter 10). The antidepressants and the calcium channel blockers may be more appropriate for the migraine patient with asthma.

Chronic Fatigue Syndrome

Chronic fatigue syndrome (CFS) has gained notoriety in last two decades, but it has been recognized for many years. The symptoms may be chronic or recurrent and include a combination of persistent and excessive fatigue, weakness, sore throat, insomnia or too much sleep, and muscular pain. Psychologic symptoms include irritability, confusion, memory loss, difficulty in concentration and thinking, and depression. Some unfortunate individuals may be disabled from this syndrome. CFS may be associated with a daily headache or, for those with a prior history of migraine, may increase the frequency and severity of the headaches. The cause of CFS has been linked to a disturbance in the immunologic system, possibly a persistent viral infection, or a masked depression. Individuals with both migraine and CFS are often greatly helped by the antidepressant drugs.

Acquired Immunodeficiency Syndrome (AIDS)

The virus that produces AIDS and AIDS-related disorders—human immunodeficiency virus (HIV)—can significantly affect the victim's nervous system. Many patients with HIV/AIDS will experience headaches—some benign and some with the same characteristics as migraine. The headaches may be generalized or on both sides, usually in the front and back of the head, and are often associated with nausea and vomiting. If the AIDS patient suffers from HIV-related meningitis, systemic infection, or a brain tumor, headache will be a prominent symptom.

If the HIV/AIDS patient is experiencing migraine, the treatment will be the same as for other migraine patients. There are other headache conditions associated with HIV/AIDS, but these disorders are beyond the scope of this book.

Renal Dialysis

Reports have documented that 70 percent of patients undergoing renal (kidney) dialysis will experience headaches. In those individuals with a prior history of migraine, the headaches will resemble a migraine attack. The headaches occur between the second and third hours of the dialysis session, and the severity is related to the duration of the interval between dialysis sessions. The dialysis headache is part of a set of symptoms—dialysis disequilibrium syndrome—which includes nausea, muscle cramping, irritability, agitation, delirium, confusion, and seizures. If the dialysis patient is also a migraine sufferer, we have to cautiously prescribe both preventative, abortive, and pain-relieving medications (chapters 9, 10, 11) in order to not impair the kidney function.

Epilepsy

For many years, epilepsy was intricately linked to migraine, particularly in children with migraine. However, the relationship between these two disorders is still undefined. Seizures may occur during a migraine aura—more often in childhood and adolescence. Rarely will patients with these seizures develop seizures unrelated to the migraine attacks. Also, headache is a common problem in the postictal period (after a seizure) for patients with epilepsy. The postictal headache develops regularly as a generalized, moderately intense, and throbbing headache. For those with both migraine and epilepsy, the migraine attacks and the postictal headache may appear identical.

Electroencephalograms (EEGs) measure brain waves, and will identify any problems in this activity. Some individuals will have abnormal EEGs throughout life but never experience a seizure. Also, migraine patients may have abnormal EEGs but these changes in brain wave patterns are not significant. In most instances, the EEGs have no relationship to the migraine.

The most recent addition to the drugs approved for the indication of migraine prevention is an anticonvulsant—divalproex sodium (commonly known as Depakote). Research is now under way in other anticonvulsant agents and their relationship to migraine. These agents are further discussed in chapter 10.

Hypertension

Migraine is not triggered by high blood pressure, but a significant number of migraine sufferers may also be suffering from hypertension. To establish a diagnosis of hypertensive headache, the diastolic pressure (the lower number of blood pressure) must be over 110 mm Hg, which represents a case of hypertension that must be treated.

To relieve this headache, the hypertension must be treated; however, coexisting hypertension may produce a challenge in migraine therapy. Older blood pressure agents, such as minoxidil and Apresoline, can trigger a migraine. Interestingly, many of the agents now used in migraine prevention were originally used for hypertension, such as the beta blockers, calcium channel blockers, and alpha agonists. These agents have a dual role—lowering

the blood pressure and preventing the migraine attacks—
and are often effective in treating both problems.

Mitral Valve Prolapse

Simply stated, mitral valve prolapse (MVP) is a common
but variable dysfunction of the mitral valve of the heart. It
is due to an excessive amount of mitral valve tissue, but the
cause is unknown. Reports have suggested that about 6
percent of the general population suffer from MVP, and it
occurs more frequently in women. Most individuals with
MVP will be asymptomatic, while others will suffer from
heart arrhythmias or chest pain below the sternum. On examination, the physician may hear a click or murmur.

It is believed that there is a high incidence of MVP
among migraine sufferers—an estimated 20 to 25 percent
of migraine victims also suffer from MVP. The basis for
the link between these two disorders is not known. Beta
blockers that also help migraine are the medications of
choice in treating MVP.

Multiple Sclerosis

Some researchers have reported that migraine headaches
were the presenting symptoms of multiple sclerosis (MS).

Also, an attack of MS may trigger headaches in those without a previous history of migraine. The actual incidence of migraine among individuals with MS has not been firmly established. These patients should be referred to a neurologist for complete evaluation and treatment.

Migraineurs with long-standing headaches will often show areas of increased intensity on MRI scanning. The uninformed practitioner who is reviewing these scans may misinterpret this finding as the beginning of MS. Treating the migraine patient with MS would be similar to standard migraine therapies.

Raynaud's Phenomenon

Raynaud's phenomenon is characterized by cold and often painful extremities because of a disorder in blood flow. This disorder occurs five times more often in women than men in the general population. However, among migraine sufferers, Raynaud's phenomenon is more prevalent in males. Its link to migraine is that both conditions are related to widening and possibly spasm of the blood vessels. The drugs usually used in migraine therapy that have an effect on the blood vessels (beta blockers, ergotamine) do not necessarily trigger this disorder. Also, drugs used to treat Raynaud's do not affect migraine treatment.

Systemic Lupus Erythematosus

Headache is a frequent initial symptom of systemic lupus erythematosus, known as SLE. SLE is a disease of the connective tissue that is progressive and can affect the skin and the lining of the blood vessels throughout the body. The headache associated with SLE is throbbing in nature and may be accompanied by scintillating scotoma (seeing bright, flashing lights), which is a common migraine aura. The migrainelike symptoms are linked to exacerbations of the SLE, rather than a coincidental occurrence. The agents of choice for SLE treatment are the corticosteroids, which are also beneficial for the headaches.

Tourette's Syndrome

Tourette's syndrome is a tic disorder that initially appears in childhood. It is characterized by multiple motor and vocal tics. Disorders that may be associated with Tourette's syndrome include obsessive-compulsive behavior, attention-deficit disorder, and other psychiatric disorders. It has been reported that there is a high incidence of migraine among both children and adults with Tourette's syndrome. Some aspects of the psychological counseling and medical treatment for Tourette's syndrome may also help the individual's migraine headaches.

Posttraumatic Migraine

Migraine attacks may follow a sudden jar or blow to the head. No matter how trivial an injury may be, an exacerbation of migraine may occur. Headache is the most dominant symptom of the postconcussion syndrome. The headache usually occurs within twenty-four hours after the injury, but could be delayed for days, weeks, and even months. The headache can be tension-type or migraine. It is possible that the head trauma may have caused the initial attack of migraine. Other symptoms of the posttraumatic syndrome are dizziness, fatigue, loss of memory, difficulty in concentration, sleep disturbances, anxiety, loss of appetite, depression, and blurred vision. The pain may be localized to the site of the trauma, and radiate to the back of the head and neck.

One example of posttraumatic migraine is "footballer's migraine." The injury occurs in soccer players who experience migraine after repeated injuries—many linked to "heading" the ball with the forehead. In addition to the headache, the individual may experience nausea, vomiting, scintillating scotoma (seeing bright, flashing light), and sensitivity to light and sound. The victim also may experience transient global amnesia, stupor, and weakness on one side of the body. Preventive treatment is similar to that described for other types of migraine in chapter 10.

Case Report

Terry Berman was a jock—during the winter he played basketball, during the spring, he was a catcher for his Little League team, and in fall he was on a traveling soccer team. Terry was now fifteen, and a high school sophomore. He had considered joining his school's football team, but he had been playing soccer since he was five, and had served on a team that won the state championship for his age group. Terry's mom and older sister had migraines, and were under my care. When he reached puberty, his mom rejoiced that it looked as if Terry wouldn't suffer from migraine. But she spoke too soon!

Terry was an all-around offensive player, and like many young soccer players, he loved to "head the ball." During the state regional tournament, Terry's team had advanced to the semis and had played against a particularly aggressive team. The headaches started the next day, along with nausea and vomiting, and some amnesia. The team trainer thought Terry had suffered a concussion. An evaluation at the local emergency department ruled out the concussion. When the headaches continued during the next week, with the associated nausea and extreme sensitivity to light, Terry's mom recognized migraine symptoms and asked me to evaluate her son.

An MRI had been performed at the emergency department and was negative. Terry's symptoms were consistent with the clinical picture of "footballer's migraine." I prescribed an NSAID for Terry for preventive therapy (see chapter 10). My plan was to switch to propranolol—a beta blocker—if Terry's headaches did not improve. However, he did well on NSAID therapy. As far as Terry's participation in athletics, I suggested that he limit his involvement in contact sports for the next few months. The last time I saw Terry, his headaches had decreased significantly (to about one every three months), and he was now playing volleyball and golf.

Injury to the neck, including whiplash, can also trigger migraine headaches. The pain may continue for several days, along with limitation of neck movement, upper back pain, and difficulty performing daily tasks. A complicated form of migraine—basilar artery migraine—may be triggered by injury to the neck.

Despite the contention of many legal experts, the recovery from posttraumatic headache is not necessarily linked to the resulting litigation. Many patients with posttraumatic syndrome will continue to have symptoms long after the lawsuits have been settled. These patients are not malingering—the headaches and other symptoms are very real.

CHAPTER 4
The Difficult Migraine Patient (Coexisting Migraine and Tension-Type Headaches)

The patient with coexisting migraine and tension-type headaches is the one most commonly seen in specialized headache clinics. Usually, these patients are suffering from daily or almost daily mild-to-moderate headaches, and another form of headache that is more severe but less frequent. The frequency of these headaches makes treatment options more complicated and also renders the individual more prone to medication-habituation problems.

Coexisting migraine and tension-type headaches are called by many names—mixed headache syndrome, chronic daily headache, or transformed migraine. Studies have shown that over one-half of migraine sufferers may also experience mild-to-moderate headaches occurring between the migraine attacks. At our clinic, I see many patients who complain of one or two migraine attacks per month but also report a daily headache. These patients complain of a continuous diffuse, dull discomfort or a constant aching pressure or tightness around the head. Some feel a sensation like insects in their scalp. Typically, the pain covers the entire head but it can be located on one side or in the frontal portion along with both sides of the head.

Clinical Features of Coexisting Migraine and Tension-Type Headaches

- A daily or almost continuous headache
- Periodic episodes of severe, one-sided, throbbing pain with some nausea and sensitivity to light
- Excessive use of ergotamines, analgesics, caffeine, or triptans
- Symptoms of anxiety or depression
- Sleep disturbance
- Family history of headaches or depression

The hard headache is typical of a migraine attack, which was described in chapter 1. The daily headache is similar to any tension-type headache, and may be described as:

- Bilateral tightness at the back of the head
- Bandlike sensations around the head
- Viselike ache
- A weight on the head
- Pressure sensation
- Soreness

The pain may be located in the forehead, temples, and/or back of the head or neck. The pain may radiate to the shoulders. Shivering or exposure to cold may exacerbate the pain. These headaches are not associated with gastrointestinal symptoms, such as nausea, vomiting, and anorexia.

Case Report

Janet Avery was a forty-three-year-old travel agent who had a long headache history dating to her adolescence. The attacks had always been intermittent until the last three years. She now had a daily headache that was continuous and always seemed to be present. About two to three times per month, she would experience her old headaches—much more painful and associated with nausea and vomiting. The daily headache was across her forehead on both sides of the head, while the hard headache was always one-sided. Janet described the daily headache as dull and annoying, but the hard headache was another story. It was totally incapacitating, and meant that she missed work and had even canceled "free" trips that she won at her agency. She was now experiencing difficulty falling asleep—she could toss and turn for one or two hours each night. When I inquired if she was anxious about anything, she stated that her oldest child was getting ready to start college and the tuition was extremely high, even with a partial scholarship. She and her husband felt they had saved enough, but with two more starting college in the next five years, Janet was panicked.

Janet occasionally had headaches at period time, but found that the hard headaches were precipitated by fatigue and missing a meal. She also consumed five to six cups of coffee per day, and when that first cup of morning coffee was delayed, she would get a hard headache. She did not notice any seasonal relationship to her headaches, nor did she notice any aura or warning symptoms of the hard headache. The daily headache was there when she awakened.

I told Janet that she was suffering from coexisting migraine and tension-type headaches. Because of the insomnia, I thought she was suffering from anxiety. Her excessive consumption of coffee was also contributing to her headache problem.

In any type of chronic tension-type headache, the daily headache is usually present in the morning when the individual awakens and he or she is typically never headache-free during the day. Many of these patients previously had intermittent headaches, and now the attacks had become daily. It is rare for the patients to experience auras with their migraine attacks, and they report few associated symptoms. However, on up to ten or fifteen days per month, these patients will describe a hard or sick headache. They can usually distinguish the hard headache from the daily headache because it is one-sided, and nausea and sometimes vomiting are associated with it. Frequently, the hard headache will also be accompanied by sensitivity to light and sound.

Coexisting migraine and tension-type headaches occur more frequently in women, as does migraine. Also, there is usually a strong family history of migraine. The development of the daily headache may take many years to evolve, although some patients can develop the daily headaches after only a year or so of experiencing infrequent migraine or monthly migraine attacks. There is a small subgroup of patients who have never suffered from intermittent migraine attacks but develop the daily headaches from the start.

Treatment

Due to the daily nature of these headaches and the fact that the treating physician will rarely obtain a history that will distinguish the individual features, these patients are not correctly diagnosed, and thus have not been treated appropriately. Patients with coexisting migraine and tension-type headaches will usually arrive at our clinic for the first time with an extensive previous medical history. They present with long lists of treating physicians, unsuccessful treatments—including traditional and alternative therapies—repeated hospital admissions, and visits to the emergency department. Their outlook varies, with some believing that they will finally be "cured" while others are skeptical of the current physician and treatment. Because they fear the pain, they heavily rely on pain relievers and sedatives.

Because of the daily pattern of their headaches, many of these patients become habituated to analgesics—both prescribed and over-the-counter (OTC). Those taking OTC analgesics often are consuming large amounts of caffeine-containing agents that cause withdrawal problems. For many years, one of the most frequently used prescription drugs used for headache contained an addicting barbiturate—butalbital. Patients with daily headaches should never use these combination agents. Patients with the chronic daily headaches will often start taking the drugs on a daily basis. Stopping the offending agent becomes very difficult with patients consuming large quantities of drugs containing caffeine or barbiturates. The habituating drug must be discontinued before effective therapy can be started. For this purpose, our patients habituated to analgesics or other headache agents such as ergotamine are admitted to the inpatient headache unit, where they can be monitored carefully for withdrawal symptoms. In my long experience dealing with these patients, it is almost impossible to discontinue the drug without hospitalization. The patients develop a rebound phenomenon from taking the drugs on a daily basis—that is, their tolerance to the drugs increases, and the medications actually contribute to the daily headaches. If a dose is missed or skipped, a headache will occur, and the drug will again be used. Recently, I have seen the triptans (sumatriptan/Imitrex, naratriptan/Amerge, rizatriptan/Maxalt, and zolmitriptan/Zomig) being used inappropriately, and it is also necessary to hospitalize these individuals. My advice to physicians that prescribe and patients that take either the ergotamines or the triptans is that they may take their maximum doses the first day of a migraine attack but must maintain a four- to five-day hiatus before using the drug again.

Not all patients with a daily headache problem take excessive amounts of medications. In some of these individuals, the migraine attacks increase for a still-unknown reason, developing into chronic daily headaches without any drug influence.

The type of sleep disturbance that the patient is experiencing will dictate the type of treatment to be selected. For patients who experience difficulty falling asleep, the headaches are related to anxiety, and an antianxiety agent will be utilized. For patients who complain of early and/or frequent awakening, the headaches are related to depression. In treating coexisting migraine and tension-type headache, I use the antidepressant agents (see chapter 10). In the patient who can distinguish their hard or sick headache from the daily headache, I do use the migraine abortive agents (chapter 9).

The patient with migraine and depression is discussed in the next chapter. There is a high proportion of migraine sufferers who also have an anxiety disorder. Anxiety often manifests as panic attacks. Some of these individuals will have phobias or generalized anxiety. Typically, the patient with chronic anxiety will describe the daily headache as annoying, and does not associate the headache with other symptoms, such as nausea and vomiting. Difficulty falling asleep is the cardinal sign of anxiety. Because these patients have a tendency to worry about everything, including their headaches, they require a great deal of reassurance. In severe cases, particularly in younger patients, there is a high incidence of suicide attempts.

CHAPTER 5
Migraine and Depression

Migraine and depression are often linked, particularly in patients with the mixed headache syndrome (see chapter 4). For migraine patients with coexisting depression, the headache often masks the underlying depression. I should also note that for almost forty years, antidepressants have been used successfully for migraine therapy. The relationship between depression and migraine is complex, and the exact mechanism by which depression causes migraine is unknown. It is assumed that depression predisposes an individual to develop headaches. In the United Kingdom, depression is the fourth most frequently diagnosed disorder, and it ranks twelfth in the United States.

The migraine patient with concomitant depression does not usually appear depressed—he or she does not have the sad mood associated with depression. So how do I identify the depression, if I am dealing with their headache problem? These patients will relate:

- Early and/or frequent awakening
- Decreased ability to concentrate
- Low energy or fatigue
- Loss of interest in pleasurable activities
- Low or no ambition
- Indecisiveness
- Poor memory

These patients may also have a variety of *physical* complaints, including:

- Shortness of breath
- Constipation
- Weight loss
- Decreased sexual drive
- Heart palpitations
- Menstrual changes

After a careful interview, the patient may reveal *emotional* complaints:

- Feelings of guilt
- Unworthiness
- Hopelessness
- Obsession over the past, present, and future

The most severe cases may reveal a basic fear of insanity, fear of physical disease or death, and may actually be considering suicide. They may note that morning is the worst time of day. The patient with migraine and depression may relate all of his or her problems to a specific event, such as an accident, surgery, or death of a family member. The event may be perceived as much more serious and out of proportion to the actual occurrence or its impact. The patient often feels weakened or maimed by the event. In some severe cases, the migraine patient may describe weeping spells preceding the migraine attack by minutes, hours, or even days.

Certain details about the headache may indicate an underlying depression. These headaches usually appear at regular intervals in relation to daily life occurring on weekends—especially Sundays—holidays, and on the first days of vacation or after exams. These headaches are worse between 4:00 P.M. to 8:00 P.M. and 4:00 A.M. to 10:00 A.M., which typifies the diurnal variation of depression (symptoms are exacerbated in morning and evening). Headaches may occur early in the morning, when the depressed patient awakens and his or her fantasies of conflict with family members or at work are manifested. The headaches may be caused by actual conflicts or by the fear that these conflicts will occur. In talking with the depressed patient, I find that the headaches often occur when the patient is in a quiet atmosphere—out of the office for a weekend and at home. The headache often coincides with interpersonal situations in which the sufferer feels compelled to appear comfortable, relaxed, and agreeable, although he or she is trying to repress resentment toward an individual he or she is expected to love or respect.

I want to emphasize that people with depressive illness may develop bodily symptoms, and conversely people with painful organic diseases tend to become depressed. It is important for the physician treating this patient to make the distinction. It should be noted that too little attention is given to the depressive aspects of chronic headache pain and its treatment. The physical complaint is so dominant that the underlying depression tends to be overlooked. First, many people with depression have a prior history of depression or a family history of it. The first symptoms of depression may have been previously observed in relatives, friends, or the person himself or herself. Many will indicate that earlier in their life they had similar symptoms.

For the treatment of depressive headache, the use of antidepressants is discussed in chapter 10. A combination of counseling and biofeedback may be considered with the use of antidepressants.

CHAPTER 6
Danger Signs of Migraine

When should a headache sufferer seek a professional consult for their headaches? Following are danger signals in headaches that may suggest the presence of serious illness, above and beyond migraine. These signals are important for all headache sufferers, even those with a prolonged history of migraine headaches:

- Headaches that do not fit a recognizable pattern or a pattern that is easily identified
- Headaches occurring for the first time in childhood or after age fifty
- Headaches occurring for the first time that rapidly increase in frequency and intensity
- The presence of neurological symptoms, such as dizziness, blurred vision, or memory loss
- A patient who feels sick or "not right" with their headaches

- Abnormal physical symptoms, for example, heart murmurs or kidney problems
- Any rigidity (stiffness) of the neck accompanying a headache may indicate an infection or inflammation of the spinal fluid
- A headache that is precipitated by any form of exertion (straining at stool, running, sexual intercourse, bending head forward)
- A headache that is progressively worsened in frequency, duration, and severity
- Headaches that have seriously impacted daily life—causing missed days at work or school, and limiting social activities

Complicated Migraine

Migraine types other than those I have previously discussed are distinguished by the complicated symptoms that accompany the headache attack. These headaches include hemiplegic migraine, ophthalmoplegic migraine, ophthalmic migraine, lower-half headache, periodic aural neuralgia, basilar artery migraine, and abdominal migraine.

Hemiplegic Migraine

A headache associated with weakness of the arm or leg on the same side affected by the headache is termed hemiplegic migraine. The symptom of weakness may appear either before the headache starts or during the acute attack, and a loss of sensory function on one side of the body may also occur. The symptoms usually disappear in a few hours or days, but in rare cases, the weakness or sensory loss is permanent.

After carefully questioning the patient, the physician often finds a previous history of this type of headache in the family—familial hemiplegic migraine. Frequently, the symptoms affect the patient on the same side of the body as it did another family member. In familial hemiplegic migraine, a genetic link has been identified.

Because hemiplegic migraine is a rare occurrence, the physician must do a thorough examination to rule out an organic cause for the headache—such as a brain tumor. Treatment, which varies according to the individual case, must be determined by a headache specialist.

Ophthalmoplegic Migraine

Ophthalmoplegic migraines are headache attacks accompanied by weakness of one or more of the eye muscles, resulting in decreased eye movement. Usually, the muscles supplied by the third cranial nerve are affected. The symptoms include drooping or swelling of the eyelid, dilation of the pupil, and double vision. Typically, ophthalmoplegic migraine appears in childhood.

The complicated manifestations are initially considered ordinary accompanying symptoms of migraine because they disappear after each headache. However, the muscle weakness and the pupil abnormality may become apparent later in life. Double vision often accompanies migraine, but if the symptom continues more than two hours, the physician must consider a problem other than migraine. Double vision and muscle weakness may be caused by an aneurysm or it may have another organic origin. As in hemiplegic migraine, the individual should undergo a thorough examination and appropriate testing to rule out conditions other than ophthalmoplegic migraine. Treatment should be determined by a headache specialist.

Ophthalmic Migraine

A distinctive type of migraine with visual symptoms is the ophthalmic migraine. It is typified by temporary blind spots, total blindness, or only seeing part of a visual field. These symptoms occur at the height of a migraine attack, rather than at the onset of the headache. Ophthalmic migraine occurs primarily in young men, who as they advance in age only suffer from the visual symptoms, not the headache. Because of the idiosyncrasies of this condition, these patients should be referred to a headache specialist.

Facial Migraine or Lower-Half Headache

This type of migraine headache is unilateral, usually starting on one side of the nose or in the palate, then radiating to the ear, cheek, or neck. It may last for several hours or even an entire day. The pain can either be a dull ache or a sharp pain. Because these patients will often experience abdominal complaints, such as nausea and vomiting, it is considered a variety of migraine. The treatment for lower-half headache is similar to that of migraine with or without aura.

Periodic Aural Neuralgia

This variety of migraine occurs at intervals, which can last for several months with attacks occurring almost daily. The pain is a severe, steady ache deep within the ear. It is accompanied by diffuse discomfort in the cheek and aching in the upper jaw. Other causes for the pain should be ruled out. The treatment should be handled by a headache specialist.

Basilar Artery Migraine

Basilar artery migraine is a severe, complicated type of migraine that is fortunately very rare. It gained its name since the blood vessel involved in this kind of headache is the basilar artery. This type of migraine is preceded by a severe dizziness, double vision, lack of coordination, fainting, or loss of consciousness. The symptoms usually disappear when the headache starts. However, the symptoms may continue for several days after the pain has disappeared. The headache itself is in the occipital region or the back of the head, affects both sides, and may radiate down into the neck, forward to the front of the head, or to the top of the head. The headache is severe and throbbing, and is usually associated with nausea, and possibly intractable vomiting. The headache rarely continues over twenty-four hours. The vomiting may be so severe that the victim becomes dehydrated.

Because this form of migraine is often seen in young women and the associated symptoms are confusion, dizziness, difficulty in coordination, its onset may suggest drug intoxication. The patient may be misdiagnosed in the emergency department and hospitalized for drug detoxification. However, a careful history will reveal that the patient, and possibly a family member, has experienced similar headaches and accompanying symptoms. A specialist should be consulted if this type of migraine is suspected.

Abdominal Migraine

This is a rare variant of migraine, in which the attacks comprise abdominal pain instead of a headache. The diagnosis is dependent on a family history of migraine because there are no abnormal physical findings. The pain may be associated with nausea and vomiting and it occurs at regular intervals.

The symptoms of abdominal migraine may be referred to as the "periodic syndrome," for a group of symptoms occurs at regular intervals. The symptoms include limb pain, abdominal pain, and headache. In children, cyclical vomiting, in which abdominal pain and vomiting occur at intervals, may be a form of abdominal migraine. Recurrent pain in their arms and legs may be described as "growing pains" and may be the only manifestation of the periodic syndrome. Many children with periodic syndrome complain of migraine attacks later in life. Treatment usually consists of anticonvulsant drugs rather than drugs normally used for migraines.

Other Alarms

Patients who maintain that their hearing becomes very acute during a migraine attack are very likely in the early stages of inner-ear disease. The patient's hearing may be very limited for faint or low-level sounds, but their perception for loud sounds may be normal or even greater than normal. This disturbance usually is present in the headache phase, but may occur as a preheadache symptom or even independently of a headache attack. During the preheadache period or the acute migraine attack, deafness may occur. Another hearing disturbance, tinnitus (persistent ringing noises in the ears or head), may occur as an aura. If this symptom continues between attacks, it may be due to an independent organic cause.

Any change in the headache pattern—increase in frequency or severity and more complex associated symptoms—should alert the migraine sufferer to seek professional help. A growing dependency or tolerance to headache drugs should also prompt a physician consultation. A long history of migraine does not render the individual free from more complicated and possibly life-threatening causes of headache.

PART II
TREATING YOUR MIGRAINE

Divinum est sedare dolorem.
(It is divine to abolish pain.)

CHAPTER 7
Self-Help Measures for Your Migraine Headaches

Migraine treatment can be divided into four phases: general (self-help) measures; abortive therapy; pain relief measures; and preventive (prophylactic) therapy. The identification and reduction of headache triggers should be the initial stage of migraine therapy. The triggers include weather changes, altitude changes, bright lights, hormones, oversleeping, excessive fatigue, missing or skipping a meal, vasoactive substances in food, alcoholic beverages, caffeine, and certain medications. Emotional provocateurs include stress, depression, anxiety, fear, and repressed hostility. Migraine sufferers may be sensitive to any, or all, of these triggers. The trigger does not necessarily precipitate a migraine each time it occurs, and it may be a combination of triggers that starts a migraine attack. The easiest way to identify headache triggers is to maintain a daily diary on which each attack is recorded, and if any trigger is associated with the attack. For women, you should also record the days of your menstrual period.

General measures for migraine treatment include:

- *Maintaining a regular sleeping schedule*

Migraine attacks may be precipitated by oversleeping or fatigue. On weekends, holidays, and during vacations, the individual may experience a migraine attack, although he or she is relaxed and does not feel tired. For these migraine sufferers, it is important to awaken at the same time each day. At our clinic, I advise the patients that on those days when they are not off to school or work, they get up at the same time as a regular school/work day and eat or drink something. If the person is so inclined, they can then return to bed and enjoy some extra sleep. As for those who suffer fatigue, the needs of each individual varies and we cannot preordain the amount of sleep each person requires. However, increasing the hours of sleep by possibly one to two hours, and then maintaining that schedule, may help relieve the headaches.

- *Maintaining a regular meal schedule*

Migraine sufferers are especially sensitive to changes in schedule. Headache attacks may be triggered by missing a meal or fasting. Meals should be consumed at the same time daily, and the patient should eat breakfast at a regular time each day to avoid the weekend or holiday migraine.

- *Diet*

As we stated earlier, migraine sufferers may be sensitive to vasoactive substances in food. Vasoactive substances gained their name by their effects on blood vessels and can precipitate a migraine attack by dilating the blood vessels. These vasoactive substances include tyramine, phenyl-ethylamine, caffeine, and nitrites.

Studies have been inconclusive on the effect of diet on migraine, but, clinically, many patients will relate their acute attacks to specific foods. All the patients at the Diamond Headache Clinic follow a diet that limits foods containing vasoactive substances (see table 7.1). An elimination diet, as explained in chapter 1, will help the migraine sufferer experiment with certain triggers, such as cheese or chocolate. If consuming a particular food item on the list will provoke a headache, then you will know to avoid it, or at least limit the quantity.

Tyramine is an amine that is found in aged or preserved foods—cheese, yogurt, pickled herring, chicken livers, red wine, canned figs, and the pods of broad beans. Phenyl-ethylamine is found in chocolate—an oft-named migraine trigger. The headache precipitated by chocolate may not develop until twenty-four hours after ingestion.

Alcoholic beverages may always trigger a migraine attack—even in small quantities. Severe intoxication with any alcoholic beverage can cause a significant increase in cerebral blood flow in the brain—and the resulting hangover headache. However, red wine contains a possible migraine trigger that is neither alcohol nor tyramine, but the complex phenol compounds (flavonoid phenols) that are found in higher concentrations in red wine than white wine.

Caffeine is often added to analgesics and other migraine remedies to enhance the effect of the other agent. However, migraine sufferers appear sensitive to consuming high quantities of caffeine in beverages and medications. A migraine attack may also occur if the individual misses his or her usual morning cup of coffee or tea, or suddenly stops drinking a cola beverage.

Nitrites are added to preserved meats to maintain their color. Sodium nitrite is found in hot dogs, bacon, ham, and salami. The headache associated with nitrite ingestion is usually bilateral, often across the front of the head, and is throbbing and may be accompanied by facial flushing.

Other substances in foods may also precipitate a migraine attack. The artificial sweetener aspartame (Nutra-Sweet) has reportedly triggered migraine attacks in sensitive individuals. Monosodium glutamate (MSG) is a flavor enhancer found in many prepared foods and Asian dishes. The Chinese restaurant syndrome is linked to this substance, and includes headache as a factor in this set of symptoms. It is important to those individuals sensitive to these triggers that they carefully read labels on food items. Aspartame is found in diet soda, but it may be used in many low-calorie food items. Customers may also request that no MSG be used in the preparation of their meals.

- *Coping strategies*

Stress may be impossible to avoid, but the patient can learn to handle stress and practice relaxation methods. The patient should learn to identify particular stressors and avoid these triggers. Progressive relaxation, breathing exercises, and biofeedback are discussed in the next chapter.

These measures should be incorporated into your daily life. They are preventive methods that need to be practiced in order to avoid attacks, and also to decrease the severity of attacks when they occur.

Table 7.1 Low-Tyramine Headache Diet

General Guidelines

- Each day eat three meals with a snack at night or six small meals spread throughout the day.
- Avoid eating high-sugar foods on an empty stomach, when excessively hungry, or in place of a meal.
- All food, especially high-protein foods, should be prepared and eaten fresh. Be cautious of leftovers held for more than one or two days at refrigerator temperature. Freezer leftovers that you want to store for more than two or three days.
- Cigarette and cigar smoke contain a multitude of chemicals that will trigger or aggravate your headache. If you smoke, make quitting a high priority. Enter a smoking cessation program.
- The foods listed in the "Use with Caution" column have smaller amounts of tyramine or other vasoactive compounds. Foods with an "✳" may contain small amounts of tyramine. Other foods in the "Use with Caution" column do not contain tyramine but are potential headache "triggers." If you are taking an MAO inhibitor (monoamine oxidase inhibitor), you should test the use of restricted foods in limited amounts.

114

- Each person may have different sensitivities to a certain level of tyramine or other vasoactive compounds in foods. If you are not on a MAO inhibitor (monoamine oxidase inhibitor), you should test the use of restricted foods in limited amounts.

Foods	Allowed	Use with Caution	Avoid
Meat, fish, poultry, eggs	Freshly purchased and prepared meats, fish, and poultry	Bacon,* sausage,* hot dogs,* corned beef,* bologna,* ham,* and luncheon meats with nitrates or nitrites added	Aged, dried, fermented, salted smoked, or pickled products Pepperoni, salami, and liverwurst
	Eggs Tuna fish, tuna salad (with allowed ingredients)	Meats with tenderizer added Caviar	Nonfresh meat or liver Pickled herring
Dairy	Milk: whole, 2 percent, or skim Cheese: American, cottage, farmer, ricotta, cream cheese (2 teaspoons) Velveeta, low-fat processed	Parmesan* or Romano* as a garnish or minor ingredient Yogurt, buttermilk, sour cream ($\frac{1}{2}$ cup per day)	Aged cheese: blue, brick, Brie, Cheddar, Swiss, Roquefort, Stilton, mozzarella, provolone, Emmentaler, etc.
Breads, cereals, pasta	Commercially prepared yeast Products leavened with baking powder: biscuits, pancakes, coffee cakes, etc.	Homemade yeast-leavened breads and coffee cake Sourdough breads	Any with restricted ingredient

Foods	Allowed	Use with Caution	Avoid
Breads, cereals, pasta (cont.)	All hot and dry cereals All pasta: spaghetti, rotini, ravioli (with allowed ingredients), macaroni, and egg noodles		
Vegetables	Asparagus, string beans, beets, carrots, spinach, pumpkin, tomatoes, squash, zucchini, broccoli, potatoes, onions cooked in food, Chinese pea pods, snow peas, navy beans, soybeans, any not on list to restrict	Raw onion	Fava or broad beans, sauerkraut, pickles, and olives Fermented soy products like miso, soy sauce, and teriyaki sauce
Fruits	Apple, applesauce, cherries, apricots, peaches, any not on restricted list	Limit intake to ½ cup per day from each group: Citrus—orange, grapefruit, tangerine, pineapple, lemon, and lime Avocados, banana, figs,* raisins,* dried fruit,* papaya, passion fruit, and red plums	
Nuts and seeds			All nuts: peanuts, peanut butter, pumpkin seeds, sesame seeds, walnuts, pecans, etc.

	Foods Allowed	Foods to Use with Caution	
Soups	Soups made from allowed ingredients, homemade broths	Canned soups with autolyzed or hydrolyzed yeast,* meat extracts,* or monosodium glutamate (MSG)	
Beverages	Decaffeinated coffee, fruit juices, club soda, caffeine-free carbonated beverages	Limit caffeinated beverages to no more than 2 servings per day: * Coffee and tea: 1 cup = 1 serving * Carbonated beverages and chocolate milk or hot cocoa: 12 ounces = 1 serving Limit alcoholic beverages to 1 serving: * 4 ounces Riesling wine, 1.5 ounces vodka or Scotch per day = 1 serving per day (May need to omit if on MAOI)	Alcoholic beverages: Chianti, Sherry, Burgundy, vermouth, ale, beer, and nonalcoholic fermented beverages; all others not specified in caution column
Desserts and sweets	Any made with allowed foods and ingredients: sugar, jelly, jam, honey, hard candies, cakes, cookies	Chocolate-based products: ice cream (1 cup), pudding (1 cup), cookies (1 average size), cakes (3-inch cube), and chocolate candies (½ ounce). (All count as 1 serving of caffeinated beverage)	Mincemeat pie

117

Foods	Allowed	Use with Caution	Avoid
Ingredients listed on food labels	Any not listed in the restricted section		MSG* (in large amounts), nitrates and nitrites (found mainly in processed meats), yeast, yeast extracts, brewer's yeast, hydrolyzed or autolyzed yeast, meat extracts, meat tenderizers Papain, bromelin, seasoned salt (containing MSG), soy sauce, teriyaki sauce
Fat, oils, and miscellaneous	All cooking oils and fats White vinegar Commercial salad dressing with allowed ingredients All spices not listed in restricted ingredients	Wine, apple, or other fermented vinegars*	Mixed dishes made with restricted ingredients: macaroni and cheese, beef Stroganoff, cheese blintzes, Asian foods, pizza Frozen entrée: read labels to check for restricted ingredients

Caffeine Content of Selected Beverages:

Carbonated beverages, 12 ounces (regular and sugar-free)	30 to 50 mg
Caffeine-free carbonated beverages	0 mg
Coffee, 6 ounces	103 mg
Decaffeinated coffee 6 ounces	2 mg
Tea, 6 ounces (instant and 3-minute brew)	31 to 36 mg

What Is Tyramine?

Tyramine is produced in foods from the natural breakdown of the amino acid tyrosine. Tyramine is not added to foods. Tyramine levels increase in foods when they are aged, fermented, stored for long periods of time, or are not fresh.

CHAPTER 8

Nondrug Treatment

For many migraine sufferers, relaxation therapy is essential for obtaining relief. Biofeedback training, relaxation exercises, and breathing exercises all can be utilized to help prevent migraine, and decrease the severity of attacks.

How Biofeedback Works

Biofeedback is a technique by which subjects can be taught to control certain functions of the autonomic (involuntary) nervous system. These functions include heart rate, blood pressure, skin temperature, muscle tension, and brain wave activity, all of which were long considered to be beyond an individual's voluntary control.

Patients learn to control these functions by observing monitoring devices and reproducing desired behavior. For example, blood pressure is monitored and the subject's goal is to learn to decrease the pressure. The blood pressure monitor advises the subject through either visual or sound feedback when the blood pressure changes. The patient then tries to consciously reproduce the conditions that caused the blood pressure to decrease.

The primary goal of biofeedback training is to provide the patient a tool with which the individual can abort and/or prevent headaches—eventually without the use of instrumentation and relying on these techniques in daily situations. The objective is to lessen the frequency, severity, and duration of headaches, and to lower or eliminate medication intake whenever possible.

Research has demonstrated the effectiveness of temperature and electromyographic (EMG) training in the treatment of migraine and tension-type headaches.

Temperature training consists of learning hand-warming techniques, in which peripheral blood flow (from the arms and legs) is redirected. Changes in the swelling or narrowing of the peripheral blood vessels produce changes in blood flow and thus have a great impact on a migraine headache. To measure if these changes in blood flow are occurring, the skin temperature is monitored. EMG training is a method of learning to achieve deep muscle relaxation in muscles that previously were thought to be beyond our voluntary control. The EMG trainer monitors muscle tension, and feeds back to the patient the amount of tension, and the amount of relaxation. The patient then learns to recognize when muscular tension begins to increase, and when and how to relax those muscles that affect headache activity.

Relaxation techniques, used during biofeedback training, are also used to control these bodily functions. They may be progressive relaxation exercises in which the subject tenses and relaxes the muscles in various parts of the body. By using these exercises, patients can identify which muscles they are tensing or when they are tensing the muscles. Other methods for relaxation include yoga and transcendental meditation. Or the subject may be successful in focusing on an image of quiet, rest, and solitude.

Biofeedback and Headache

The use of biofeedback in headache was suggested initially in the early 1970s by the work of Dr. Elmer Green of the Menninger Foundation. In conducting biofeedback research with volunteer subjects, Dr. Green noted that one of his subjects initially experienced difficulty increasing the skin temperature of her hand during a migraine attack. However, the headache was terminated when she was finally able to increase her hand temperature. Thereafter, she focused on warming her hands whenever she experienced a migraine attack, finding a technique that stopped the headache from progressing and decreasing the need for medications. Dr. Green, along with Dr. Joseph Sargent and E. Dale Walters, then instituted a study utilizing headache patients. These patients were instructed to raise their hand temperatures by employing phrases that focus on warmth and relaxation. The temperature was monitored using a thermometer taped to the subject's dominant index finger. Thus, the subject would be able to observe any increase in hand temperature. At the time of an acute headache, the subject would employ these techniques in the hope of stopping the headaches. It should be noted that the researchers also tried taping the thermometer to the subject's forehead and asked the subject to cool the area. This process was not successful—the only significant results occurred when the subjects tried to warm their hands. Why the hands? It was simple to focus on the hand and easier to measure the finger temperature.

About the time Dr. Green and his associates were conducting the temperature feedback studies, Drs. Thomas Budzynski, Johannes Stoyva, and Charles Adler were studying the effects of deep muscle relaxation measured by an EMG monitor. The forehead muscle tension was monitored and was fed back to the subject by a tone. As the muscle tension increased, the tone increased, and vice versa. By using relaxation techniques (progressive relaxation exercises, listening to relaxing music, or focusing on relaxing subjects), the subject was able to decrease the tension across the forehead. The researchers then employed these techniques on patients with tension-type (muscle contraction) headaches. The patients learned to decrease the muscle tension in their foreheads, and also noted a decrease in the frequency and severity of their headaches.

Temperature Training

At the Diamond Headache Clinic, patients initially start temperature training with an orientation session, consisting of a twenty-minute period limited to temperature training techniques. The patient is positioned in a comfortable recliner chair, and a thermometer is attached with paper tape to the tip of the index finder on the dominant hand. The lights in the treatment room are dimmed, and soft ocean sounds are played. During this session, the goals of biofeedback training are explained, as well as the basic instructions for the training. For home use, patients are provided a monitor that measures the surface temperature—a simple thermometer that the patient can easily read. In order to increase the hand temperature, the patient is provided a set of phrases that focuses on warmth and is also relaxing. The patient will also be instructed on diaphragmatic breathing, which is discussed later in this chapter.

At the next visit, usually one week later, the biofeedback technician will proceed with the temperature training. Then, the patient is instructed to imagine the sights, smells, sounds, and touch sensations of a beach scene. The technician will describe the scene in detail as the ocean tape plays. This procedure can last anywhere from ten to thirty minutes, depending on the patient's success in learning. The patient is then instructed to imagine herself in this scene, lying on a favorite blanket or towel on the beach. The imagery will then lead into specific images:

"Imagine the sun is warming the face, the hands, the feet. Feel the warmth of the sun. Imagine dipping your hands into the warm sand . . . ," etc. (In one case, at the initial temperature feedback training session, the patient was able to increase the hand temperature from 86.8 degrees Fahrenheit to 91.7 degrees Fahrenheit—a 4.9 degree difference.) After this exercise, the patient will be advised to slowly remove himself or herself from the scene and will be asked to stretch in order to focus on the session once more. The patient will be shown a detailed graph of the minute-by-minute temperature changes, and encouraged to continue the imagery exercise twice daily while attached to the temperature training unit.

The speed at which the patient increases the hand temperature is very important so that the patient may utilize these techniques at the first symptoms of a headache. If the techniques are used immediately, the headache may be stopped.

Patients are instructed to practice these exercises at least twice daily. They are provided the thermometers in order to observe their progress. Patients are also encouraged to use these skills at the onset of a headache. The thermometers can be obtained from biofeedback training centers—but should be used in conjunction with a training program.

Temperature Training Phrases

These are known as autogenic phrases and were formulated by Dr. Johannes Schulz. You will note that by repeating these phrases, it is hoped that you will become relaxed, and also increase the temperature of your hands (as you are really increasing the blood flow to your hands). Remember: You are in charge of this training—you are in the "driver's seat."

I feel quiet. . . . I am beginning to feel quite relaxed. . . . My feet feel heavy and relaxed. . . . My ankles, my knees, and my hips feel heavy, relaxed, and comfortable. . . . My solar plexus and the whole central portion of my body feel relaxed and quiet. . . . My hands, my arms, and my shoulders feel heavy, relaxed, and comfortable. . . . My neck, my jaws, and my forehead feel relaxed, they feel comfortable and smooth. . . . My whole body feels quiet, heavy, comfortable, and relaxed. I am quite relaxed. . . . My arms and hands are heavy and warm. . . . I feel quiet. . . . My whole body is relaxed and my hands are warm. . . . My hands are warm. . . . Warmth is flowing into my hands. . . . They are warm. . . . warm.

EMG Feedback Training

At our clinic, the patient is then instructed on the biofeedback method of EMG techniques. At the first session, electrodes are placed on the patient's forehead. You will be familiar with an electrode if you have ever had an electrocardiogram (EKG). They are round or square disks that are usually applied to the body with some type of adhesive. With EMG training, the electrodes can be placed at different sites of the body—wherever the tension is located. With most headache patients, it is easier to start relaxing the forehead muscles. The patient will receive feedback about the tension via an audio signal—typically, an annoying sound. Until the patient is able to completely relax the frontalis muscle, the tone continues. The reward occurs when the annoying sound turns off due to the relaxation of the forehead. The patient will then be asked to continue diaphragmatic breathing as the technician speaks in a soft, even tone.

The instructions heard by the patient follow:

Let all your muscles go loose and heavy. Settle back quietly and comfortably. As you breathe in, imagine clean, fresh air cleansing out the body. Your stomach rises as you breathe in, falls as you breathe out. Let the air clean out all of the tension that you have in your body. Blow out all of the tension and pain, blow it out and away. Your tummy is simply rising and falling with air. Allow your body to pause as you exhale all of the air in your lungs. Start up again only when you need to. Notice the sound on the machine is getting lower and lower in tone, you are doing well. Now imagine warmth and heaviness spreading over your scalp. Your scalp feels loose and heavy. Let your forehead become loose and heavy. Allow all the muscles in your temples to become heavy and

127

warm, release your lower jaw. All of your facial muscles feel smooth and heavy, as your tummy rises and falls with air. You are starting to feel warm and heavy all over, all over your head and face. You feel quiet and calm, but are still alert. Notice the sound on the machine has turned off; it only beeps a little now. Now let's relax the throat muscles. . . .

The EMG training session will continue for twenty minutes, and often the patient will exhibit a gradual decline of forehead muscle tension. The patient will be instructed to use the home thermal training unit at least twice before the next appointment. Each patient is provided a set of biofeedback exercises to practice independently.

If necessary, we will encourage the patient to work at reducing the tension in other muscle groups, such as the shoulder muscles. For example, for patients who are students or office workers, who are usually sitting at a desk, biofeedback training may be undertaken with the individual sitting in an upright chair for the sessions focusing on relaxing the neck and shoulder muscles. Our purpose for this type of training is to help the patient incorporate these exercises into their daily routine. Focusing on posture is another tool to help the patient achieve more relaxed neck and shoulder muscles.

During EMG biofeedback training, the patient may identify common physical signs of stress, such as:

- Teeth grinding
- Jaw clenching

- Tightening of the forehead
- Wrinkling of the brow
- Obvious tension in the neck
- Tightening of the shoulders

By learning to relax these stress points at times of stress or stop tensing these areas at the onset of a headache, or at bedtime, the patients may notice a decrease in the severity of the headache attacks. We encourage the patient to practice the progressive relaxation exercises listed below.

The usual training period is four weeks, with follow-up sessions scheduled according to the patient's progress. Patients are encouraged to continue twice-daily practice.

However, patients habituated to analgesics are usually not successful with biofeedback training until they have been successfully weaned from these drugs. Children with headaches are excellent candidates for biofeedback training. They are more receptive to learning new techniques and have not learned the pain behavior so often seen in adult headache patients. In other words, these children do not have a secondary gain from their headaches. Too often, patients learn that they can gain attention or avoid people and situations that bother them by complaining of a headache.

It is hoped that by utilizing the biofeedback training techniques, patients will be able to control the frequency and severity of their headaches. They also may be able to decrease the amount of pain medication taken and eventually discontinue all medications.

Progressive Relaxation Exercises

These exercises, used in EMG feedback training, were developed by Dr. Joseph Wolpe to teach the subject to recognize the difference between tense and relaxed muscles. The complete list includes relaxing the entire body. However, in treating headache patients, we focus on the upper part of the body. In these exercises, the concept is one of instruction—you are being given direction. For some patients, taping these exercises—in their own voice—is most helpful. Other patients may find it more relaxing to listen to someone with a soft, soothing voice to present these exercises.

Let all your muscles go loose and heavy. Just settle back quietly and comfortably. . . . Wrinkle up your forehead now; wrinkle and smooth it out. Picture the entire forehead and scalp becoming smoother as the relaxation increases. . . . Now frown and crease your brows and study the tension. . . . Let go of the tension again, smooth out the forehead once more. . . . Now, close your eyes tighter and tighter. Feel the tension. . . . Now relax your eyes. Keep your eyes closed, gently, comfortably, and notice the relaxation. . . . Now clench your jaws. Bite your teeth together; study the tension throughout the jaws. . . . Relax your jaws now. Let your lips part slightly. . . . Appreciate the relaxation. Now press your tongue hard against the roof of your mouth. Look for the tension. . . . All right, let your tongue return to a comfortable and relaxed position. . . . Now purse your lips, press your lips together tighter and tighter. . . . Relax the lips. Note the contrast between tension and relaxation. Feel the relaxation all over your face, all over your forehead and scalp, eyes, jaws, lips, tongue, and your neck muscles. . . . Press your head back as far as it can go and feel the tension shift. . . . Now roll it to the left. . . . Straighten your head and bring it forward and press your chin against your chest. Let your head return to a comfortable position, and study the relaxation. Let the relaxation develop. Shrug your shoulders right up. Hold the tension. . . . Drop your shoulders and feel the relaxation. Neck and shoulders are relaxed. . . . Shrug your shoulders again and move them around. Bring your shoulders up and forward and back. Drop your shoulders once more and relax. Let the relaxation spread deep into the shoulders, right into your back muscles. Relax your neck and throat, and your jaws and other facial areas as the pure relaxation takes over and grows deeper . . . deeper . . . ever deeper.

Which Method Is Right for You?

In treating headache patients with biofeedback, the appropriate method must be selected. Patients whose only headaches are migraines may be helped with temperature feedback training only, but the combination of EMG and temperature feedback training is preferred for most headache patients. Patients with tension-type (muscle contraction) headaches would not be successfully treated with temperature training alone, but these patients could be treated exclusively with EMG feedback.

An important factor in biofeedback training is placing the responsibility for therapy with the individual; the physician or therapist merely serves as a teacher. It is essential for the success of the training that the patient thoroughly practice all pertinent techniques.

Diaphragmatic Breathing

At the first visit in the biofeedback area, following EMG training, the patient will be instructed in the methods of diaphragmatic breathing. Typically, the technician working with the patient will first demonstrate this breathing method, explaining that in order to develop the relaxation response, the largest part of the lung capacity will be used. The diaphragm expands as the patient breathes in, allowing the largest portions of the lungs to fill. The diaphragm relaxes as she exhales, thereby the "stomach" will fall on this exhalation. During this exercise, the patient is using the highest percentage of oxygen to travel into the bloodstream, the bloodstream into the muscle, and then the muscles loosening. The patient will be asked if she is feeling more relaxed with each breath; the reply is usually "Yes." After learning the breathing technique, the technician will place one of the patient's hands on the stomach so that his or her progress can be easily monitored. The correct diaphragmatic breathing technique often becomes a favorite technique for our patients.

Patterns of breathing can signal and trigger specific responses of the nervous system. The appropriate use of diaphragmatic breathing can help the individual correct emergency stress responses. The emergency response of "fight or flight" is similar to the idea of "survival of the fittest"—allowing for instantaneous heightening of the senses and strength for survival under life-threatening conditions. However, this response may be overused in an environment in which nonphysical stress often permeates all aspects of life. Therefore, the mind must adapt many problem-solving patterns, and too often these patterns become dysfunctional and result in inappropriate physical responses, such as headache, sleep disturbance, or gastrointestinal disorder (ulcer, colitis).

Early recognition of this phenomenon and the use of correct diaphragmatic breathing techniques are also powerful tools in reversing dysfunctional automatic responses to stress that can trigger and exacerbate headache. The breathing techniques are the natural way to breathe, best observed in an infant's breathing patterns. Dysfunctional breathing patterns are often formed through unconscious learning.

It is hoped that the patients will be able to recognize the correlation between cold hands and stress and/or headache (all signals for the "fight or flight" response), as well as the effects of diaphragmatic breathing. We also strive for the patients to experience a relaxation response. Through this training, we hope that the patient will respond to stress in a more effective, controlled manner.

Diaphragmatic Breathing Exercises

The following breathing exercises are designed to help you achieve the relaxation response. These exercises should be done many times a day (especially when stress levels are high) to help relieve tension and pain, as well as to clear the mind.

General Practice Information

All breathing exercises should be done by taking slow, gentle, deep breaths. All breathing exercises are to be done diaphragmatically, that is to say, using the diaphragm and not the shoulders and chest. This is easily accomplished by the use of the abdominal muscles in the following way:

- When exhaling, always contract (pull in) the abdomen.
- When inhaling, always distend (push out) the abdomen.

It is helpful to practice this before going on to the breathing exercises themselves.

Breathing exercises should be done in a slow, evenly flowing process, paying special attention to making the transition between inhalation and exhalation smooth and even. Begin all breathing exercises by exhaling all air out of your lungs and pulling in the abdomen at the same time.

Exercise 1

- Exhale completely, pulling in the abdominal muscles.

- Begin a low, gentle inhalation through the nose while slowly and simultaneously distending the abdomen. Imagine that you are breathing in a sense of easy, quiet energy and well-being. Take this breath down to the bottom of your lungs, allowing your chest to expand slightly. Do not allow your shoulders to rise.

- When your lungs feel full, allow a slow, smooth transition between inhaling and exhaling.

- Begin to exhale through your mouth slowly, while contracting the abdominal muscles, again remembering not to move your shoulders. While exhaling, imagine that you are bringing up from within you any discomfort and muscle tension with your breath.

- Blow your breath gently away from you through your mouth, allowing a sense of quiet to take over your body.

- Repeat the above three steps twice more.

Exercise 2

- Exhale completely, pulling in the abdominal muscles.

- Take a slow, deep "tummy" breath and, as you inhale, say the number five to yourself.

- Exhale slowly, fully; put your hand on your stomach and watch it.

- Say the number four to yourself and inhale.

- As you exhale, say to yourself, "I am more relaxed now than I was at number five." Be sure not to rush the thought.

- Say the number three to yourself while inhaling.

- As you exhale, say to yourself, "I am more relaxed now than I was at number four."

- Continue this process until you have counted down to the number one.

Exercise 3

- Exhale completely, pulling in the abdominal muscles. Imagine that your lungs are divided horizontally into three parts.

- Take a deep "tummy" breath. Visualize the lowest part of your lungs filled with air. Use only your diaphragm; your chest and shoulders remain still.

- Imagine the middle part of your lungs filling with air and, as you visualize the expansion, allow your rib cage to expand.

- Visualize the upper part of your lungs filling with air and your lungs becoming completely filled. Allow your shoulders to rise slightly.

- Slowly begin to exhale, allowing your shoulders to drop slightly. Visualize the air leaving the top portion of your lungs.

- Visualize the air leaving the middle portion of your lungs and feel your rib cage contract.

- Pull in your abdomen to force out the last bit of air from the bottom of your lungs.

- Repeat the exercise three times.

Imagery

The use of imagery or visualization to affect changes in responding to stress is a concept that has been used for centuries, and has not been limited to medicine. Imagery has been utilized in the arts, religion, philosophy, and many other fields. It is a basic process of the mind, and a basic element of thought. Scientists have found that responses to stress can be triggered by visualizing an activity, such as when confronting simulated stimuli from the external world. An individual will respond with many of the same physical changes in facing a "hungry tiger" as to imagining a frightening creature lurking behind a nearby door.

Sophisticated protocols using imagery were used by such notables as Sigmund Freud and Carl Jung. Today, patients are instructed to imagine or visualize a very pleasant, quiet, calming scene—one that will produce a sense of well-being and warmth, such as a sunny beach, sitting by a fireplace, or a particularly comfortable room. The scene is to be experienced using all of the senses.

With younger patients, we may use different imagery, depending on the patient's age and interests. For example, when working with a twelve-year-old boy, they found that he reacted well to imaginative settings such as ocean floors, magical forests, etc., and that he did extremely well on his own—using his own imaginative techniques of relaxing. This particular patient was encouraged to use imagery during his sessions, and he was encouraged to use these techniques in both standing and sitting positions. He reported that he had continued success with relaxation techniques, temperature training, and diaphragmatic breathing. "I use the hand stuff the most—but I also know that I have to relax and breathe when I stress out." He uses the training at the first sign of a headache, but will also use the self-regulation techniques on a daily basis to help manage stress and anxiety.

Particularly helpful tools are the visual prompts such as placing signs or labels to remind the patient to relax. For example, the young man was given "green dots" to use at home, where he applied the stickers everywhere, including the front door and the bathroom! "I put the green dots you gave me everywhere to remind me to breathe and not stress out," he stated. This young patient was enthusiastic about biofeedback, and expressed a real desire to use the techniques to help his headaches. He experiences only mild headaches once a week, and is able to stop them with biofeedback.

Imagery Techniques

The mind is a very powerful tool in the process of relaxation. A thought can elicit a physiological response. For instance, picture a lemon. In your mind go through the process of touching it, slicing it, smelling it, than taking a taste of it. This image will often make you salivate, even pucker.

You can put this valuable phenomenon to use in bringing about relaxation. By simply allowing your mind to imagine some very pleasant, quiet, calming scene, you can produce the physical responses that would be present in those surroundings. The imagined place can be either a real one that you find particularly pleasant or one conjured up in your imagination. In either case, you should imagine a place that gives you a sense of well-being and warmth. Examples:

- A sunny beach—warm sand, hot sun
- Sitting in front of a fireplace
- Holding a cup of hot coffee/tea
- Sitting in a warm tub

Before beginning the exercise, take three deep and slow breaths. Move yourself into the picture that you are imagining. Try to see, hear, smell, and feel every detail of the image as though you were there. Bring your senses close to the details of the image. Experience as much of the image as possible. Get involved in the process of being there. Continue this process for about twenty to thirty minutes.

At the end of the exercise, take two deep, slow breaths, exhaling any tension that might be left, inhaling a sense of well-being and energy.

Physical Therapy

In headache treatment, physical therapy is sometimes beneficial as an adjunctive therapy. The following physical therapy interventions are used in headache therapy:

- Deep heat to whatever location the pain is, or any area where muscles may be tense

- Massage—whatever area is particularly tense, and to relax the patient in general

- Exercise—depends on the individual; ranges from walking, treadmill, stationary bikes to aerobics. In addition to promoting health, establishing an exercise routine is another method of teaching a headache patient to have constructive activities when not in pain.

- Cold packs for acute headache—the patient may use commercially available cold packs or ordinary ice bags as "cold compresses." The use of cold may ease the decrease of the blood flow to the locale of the headache.

CHAPTER 9
Miracle Drugs of the Twenty-first Century and How They Stop Your Migraine Attack

In the past decade, enormous gains have been made in abortive therapy. In addition to the introduction of the triptan agents, newer methods of delivery for older, standard medications have greatly expanded available treatment options. The use of these newer agents has also decreased the disability associated with migraine and improved the quality of life for the migraine sufferer.

During the past three decades, research has suggested a relationship between serotonin (5-HT) and migraine. Serotonin is a chemical (or sometimes referred to as a hormone) that is primarily released by the platelets into the blood. Depending on its concentration, serotonin can control blood vessels. One theory suggests that migraine attacks are triggered by the release of serotonin from the platelets. Another theory indicates that the release of serotonin from certain nerve fibers initiates the acute attack, while another theory associates changes in serotonin metabolism as playing a role in migraine occurrence. Serotonergic drugs are medications that enhance or decrease the amount of serotonin and/or serotonin's actions. These drugs include reserpine (used for hypertension), which is a known precipitator of migraine attacks.

Agents recognized as serotonin agonists include the triptans (sumatriptan, naratriptan, zolmitriptan, rizatriptan), ergotamine, and dihydroergotamine (DHE). The triptans are a group of drugs that work on the blood vessels and the receptors, which are like switching stations that control blood vessel action. These drugs may have specific effects on areas of the brain that also control select blood vessels. The triptans have demonstrated efficacy in stopping migraine attacks by appearing to affect the serotonin receptors. These agents also block inflammation—which is believed to be the cause of migraine pain. In addition to these actions, sumatriptan can produce narrowing of blood vessels in the brain that are widened during an acute migraine attack.

The Triptans

Sumatriptan Succinate

Sumatriptan, commonly known as Imitrex, was the first triptan to be approved for migraine abortive therapy. Unlike the ergot preparations (described later in this chapter), sumatriptan has been effective in many cases, even in

the advanced stages of a migraine attack. When first introduced, sumatriptan was only available for subcutaneous injections, which are directly under the skin. Sumatriptan is
now available for oral or intranasal administration.

Sumatriptan is usually well tolerated with minor side
effects such as flushing, tingling, neck or chest tightness or
pain, nausea, and throat discomfort. If the first dose of
sumatriptan offers at least partial headache relief, a second
dose may be repeated after an hour, or any time within the
next twenty-four hours if the headache recurs. However, a
five-day hiatus should be maintained between days of use.
Sumatriptan should not be used in patients with basilar or
hemiplegic migraine, ischemic heart disease, or Prinzmetal's angina, and cannot be used if you are also taking
ergot-containing preparations or monoamine oxidase inhibitors (MAOIs) (discussed in chapter 10).

Naratriptan

Naratriptan, commonly known as Amerge, is a second-
generation 5-HT agonist. It remains active in the blood
vessels for a longer interval (six hours) than the other triptans and may be the best choice if you experience migraine
recurrence and menstrual migraine. It has a low incidence
of side effects, with the most frequent being nausea and
vomiting. This drug is available for oral administration.
Naratriptan should not be used in patients with ischemic
heart disease, Prinzmetal's angina, or in patients with basi-

lar or hemiplegic migraine. Naratriptan cannot be used if you are also taking an ergot-containing preparations or MAOIs.

Zolmitriptan

Zolmitriptan, commonly known as Zomig, is absorbed quickly, and faster resolution of the migraine attack may be observed with its use. This drug also appears effective in managing the associated symptoms of migraine, including nausea and sensitivity to light and sound. This medication reduced the disability associated with migraine. Its side effects are similar to sumatriptan, with the most frequently reported symptoms including nausea, dizziness, prickling or tingling of the skin, drowsiness, warm or cold sensations, jaw pain, and tightness of the neck or throat. Zolmitriptan is available as an oral tablet. This medication should not be used in patients with basilar or hemiplegic migraine, ischemic heart disease, or Prinzmetal's angina. Zolmitriptan cannot be used if you are taking ergot-containing preparations or MAOIs.

Rizatriptan

Rizatriptan, commonly known as Maxalt, is also absorbed rapidly, and in studies its effects were noted within thirty minutes of ingestion. This agent is well tolerated, and the most commonly reported side effects are bitter taste, dizziness, tiredness, sleepiness, and nausea. It is available as an oral tablet as well as a disk for oral disintegration—that means it can be taken without water. Similar to the other triptans, this drug cannot be used in patients with basilar or hemiplegic migraine, ischemic heart disease, or Prinzmetal's angina. Also, it cannot be given if you are using ergot-containing preparations or MAOIs.

Ergotamine Tartrate

Before the introduction of sumatriptan (Imitrex), the drug most commonly used to abort the acute attack was ergotamine tartrate. It was first introduced for migraine therapy about fifty years ago. In addition to its decreasing serotonin activity, ergotamine acts directly to narrow blood vessels, counteracting the widening of the blood vessels in the brain, which causes the pain.

In the United States, ergotamine is only available for sublingual (under the tongue) administration (Ergomar) or combined with caffeine in an oral tablet (Wigraine and Ercaf). To be effective, ergotamine tartrate must be taken as soon as the symptoms of an attack appear. Patients with migraine with aura should take the ergotamine as soon as the aura starts.

Caution should be used with ergotamine. The side effects include nausea, vomiting, diarrhea, cramping, dizziness, and more serious symptoms such as numbness and high blood pressure. Because of the effects of ergotamine in the blood vessels, this drug should not be used in those with a history of cardiac problems, thrombophlebitis, severe hypertension (high blood pressure), kidney or liver disease, and recent infection, and must be monitored carefully when used in those with peptic ulcer. It should never be used during pregnancy.

Excessive use of ergot can cause a phenomenon termed ergotism, a serious decrease in the circulation of the extremities. Ergot should not be taken on a daily basis or the patient may suffer from rebound headaches. If the patient continues to take the ergotamine tartrate on a daily basis because it relieves the headaches, he or she will build tolerance to the medication, and will likely take increasing amounts of the drug. Eventually, the ergots start causing the headaches. It is very difficult to treat these patients until they have stopped the ergots.

Dihydroergotamine Mesylate

Dihydroergotamine mesylate (DHE) is a derivative of ergotamine and has recently been "rediscovered" as a 5-HT receptor agonist. It, too, has been used safely and effectively in the abortive therapy of migraine for over fifty years. Unlike ergotamine tartrate, DHE is associated with less nausea and constricts the veins more than the arteries. DHE can also be used to help withdraw—"detox"—patients who are ergotamine-dependent.

The route of administration is important in obtaining relief because it impacts on the speed of action. Although oral use of any agent is the simplest route, it may not be the best method of administration in the 70 percent of migraine sufferers who experience associated nausea and vomiting. Injections offer the quickest action, but self-injection techniques may not be the patient's first choice. Until recently, DHE was only available as an injection, commonly known as D.H.E. 45. However, many patients do not tolerate self-injections, or the attack would be firmly established before the migraine victim could visit the physician's office or emergency department to receive an injection. DHE is now available as a nasal spray, commonly known as Migranal. In patients with intractable migraine—that is, migraine difficult to relieve—DHE may be given in repetitive doses intravenously, in combination with an antinausea drug, metoclopramide, commonly known as Reglan.

Due to its actions in narrowing blood vessels, DHE should not be used in individuals with peripheral vascular disease, ischemic heart disease, Prinzmetal's angina, uncontrolled hypertension, complicated migraine, impaired liver or kidney function, and infection. It should never be used during pregnancy. DHE should not be used if you also are taking the triptans or ergotamine preparations.

Isometheptene Mucate

In patients who cannot tolerate ergotamine or DHE, and in those who should not use these drugs, a drug combining isometheptene mucate, dichloralphenazone (a mild sedative), and acetaminophen may be effective. This combination drug is commonly known as Midrin. Similar to ergotamine, isometheptene narrows those widened blood vessels that cause migraine pain. It is especially beneficial for those with mild-to-moderate migraine attacks if taken early during the headache. This agent can also be used on the second or third days of a migraine attack—during that interval when the triptans, ergots, or DHE cannot be repeated. Isometheptene mucate must not be used by patients with uncontrolled hypertension, organic heart disease, or severe cases of liver or kidney disease. It should never be used in patients on MAOIs.

Nonsteroidal Anti-Inflammatory Drugs (NSAIDs)

The NSAIDs have been used successfully in migraine abortive therapy. They stabilize proteins and inhibit inflammation. For migraine abortive therapy, the NSAIDs that have been used include naproxen sodium, which is available over-the-counter as Aleve and by prescription as Anaprox or Naprelan. Other over-the-counter NSAIDs

are aspirin, ibuprofen (available as Motrin and Advil), and ketoprofen, which is marketed as Orudis. Unfortunately, the NSAIDs have a great capacity for gastrointestinal symptoms, including bleeding, and should be avoided in patients with peptic ulcer disease. Their side effects include nausea, abdominal distress, heartburn, diarrhea, dizziness, and ringing in the ears (tinnitus). The NSAIDs should not be used in patients with kidney dysfunction.

Phenothiazines

The phenothiazines are known for their sedative and antinauseant effects. Also, they may have other actions that help stop an acute migraine attack. Two of these drugs—chlorpromazine, commonly known as Thorazine, and prochlorperazine, commonly known as Compazine—have been used effectively in emergency departments for the abortive treatment of acute migraine.

Intranasal Lidocaine

A recent report has suggested the use of intranasal lidocaine, also known as Xylocaine, as a viable agent for the abortive treatment of an acute migraine attack. Relapse was common and occurred early after treatment.

Pain Relief

Complete resolution of a migraine attack may not be achieved by the abortive drugs that we have already discussed, and analgesics (pain relievers) may be helpful to eliminate the acute pain. Over-the-counter (OTC) agents can be used, including aspirin, acetaminophen (commonly known as Tylenol), ibuprofen (available as Advil or Motrin), naproxen sodium (available OTC as Aleve), and ketoprofen (commonly known as Orudis).

Aspirin, Acetaminophen, and Caffeine

A combination of aspirin, acetaminophen, and caffeine—commonly known as Excedrin Migraine—was the first OTC pain reliever to receive approval from the Food and Drug Administration for the indication of migraine pain relief. This combination agent is suggested for the acute treatment of mild-to-moderate headache without associated vomiting and disability. Recently, a preparation of ibuprofen, commonly known as Motrin Migraine or Advil Migraine, has also received approval for the indication of migraine pain relief.

Overconsumption of these analgesics, particularly OTC analgesics containing caffeine, can produce serious side effects. Withdrawal from caffeine-containing drugs may trigger the caffeine-withdrawal headache. These drugs should be avoided in those patients with frequent migraine attacks.

Other pain-relief measures for the acute migraine attacks include the narcotic analgesics, antinauseants, and cold packs. An injectable preparation of a prescription NSAID, ketorolac—commonly known as Toradol—is available. Ketorolac is advantageous because it is nonhabituating or addicting, and has a low side-effect profile. It is also available as an oral tablet.

Narcotic Analgesics

The use of the narcotic analgesics—that is, the pain relievers that contain an opiate—are usually used as injectable agents, and will provide pain relief. As with other pain syndromes, these drugs should not be used in patients with frequently occurring migraine attacks as they can become addicting. Narcotic analgesics used in relief of acute attacks include:

- Codeine
- Meperidine—commonly known as Demerol
- Methadone—commonly known as Dolophine
- Butorphanol—commonly known as Stadol

Butorphanol was originally only available as an injectable preparation. However, since the introduction of butorphanol as a nasal spray, it has been used frequently for migraine pain relief. As it's quickly absorbed via the nasal passages, and because the nasal passages have a large amount of blood vessels surrounded by very thin walls, nasal sprays can be quickly absorbed. It is an excellent pain reliever for intermittent attacks. However, we caution that frequent use of butorphanol can lead to habituation.

Antiemetics (Antinauseants)

Due to the symptoms associated with an acute migraine attack—nausea and vomiting—the antiemetics are used for injection (parenterally) or as rectal suppositories. The sedative effects of the phenothiazines are also useful for relieving the multiple symptoms present during an acute migraine attack. The phenothiazines used for migraine relief include:

- Promethazine—commonly known as Phenergan
- Chlorpromazine
- Prochlorperazine

Antiemetics that won't make you as drowsy as those drugs listed above include trimethobenzamide (commonly known as Tigan) and metoclopramide (commonly known as Reglan).

Metoclopramide is an antiemetic and also a 5-HT receptor agonist. It has been shown to enhance the absorption of oral medications and has been used effectively in combination with intravenous DHE. This drug will occasionally cause nervousness and tremor.

Cold Packs

Cold packs have been used for many years by migraine patients. The use of ice bags or commercially manufactured ice packs, along with pressure, may reduce the pulsating pain associated with acute migraine attacks. Typically, the ice is applied on the site of the pain. Or the patient may place the ice bag at the top of his or her head—whatever works best. Some patients may place ice on top of the head, and a warm compress such as a heating pad at the neck for relief of the muscles tightening because of the headache.

CHAPTER 10
Preventive Therapy of Migraine

Preventive (prophylactic) therapy should be considered in those patients experiencing two or more migraine attacks per month. This form of therapy is also recommended for patients whose attacks are severe enough to greatly impact their quality of life and ability to function, for whom abortive therapies have been unsuccessful, or for whom abortive therapies cannot be used.

In treating the patient with migraine, the patient and the physician should not be frustrated because a medication did not stop the attacks from occurring. Several trials of preventive drugs may be needed before finding the right one. These preventive drugs have significant potential for reducing the frequency, duration, and intensity of acute migraine attacks, and can be instrumental in decreasing the disability associated with chronic migraine. The treatment trials should be sufficiently long (if tolerated) to ensure that the acceptable "therapeutic" levels have been achieved. However, the trials should be short enough to avoid prolonged courses of noneffective medications. A time frame for these treatment intervals of approximately four to six weeks is reasonable but may differ according to the medicine chosen and the individual response time of the patient. Beyond this period, if patients do not report improvement, another medication should be tried.

Four agents have been approved by the Food and Drug Administration for the indication of migraine prevention: propranolol, timolol, divalproex sodium, and methysergide.

Propranolol

Propranolol, commonly known as Inderal, is a beta blocker that is considered to be the drug of choice in migraine prevention. Beta blockers perform many activities that may contribute to their efficacy in migraine prevention, including: (1) preventing widening of the cranial arteries because they block the beta receptors; (2) blocking the platelet from clumping; and (3) decreasing the ability of platelets to stick to the walls of the smallest blood vessels—the capillaries. Propranolol was first approved for the treatment of high blood pressure (hypertension) and heart arrhythmias, and it is especially helpful for migraine sufferers who also suffer from these disorders. Propranolol is also helpful for patients with severe hypertension, angina, and prior histories of heart attacks who are not able to take ergot preparations. The patient on propranolol should be examined at regular intervals to monitor blood pressure and pulse.

At the Diamond Headache Clinic, I prefer the long-acting form of propranolol known as Inderal LA, which is easy for the patient who prefers to only take the medication once daily. The most common side effects include fatigue, gastrointestinal disturbances, insomnia, nightmares, hypotension (low blood pressure), cold extremities, decreased resting heart rate, and sexual dysfunction. The drug is not recommended in patients with asthma, chronic obstructive lung disease, congestive heart failure, atrioventricular conduction disturbances, or in patients receiving treatment with insulin, oral hypoglycemic (antidiabetic) drugs, or MAOIs. Because the drug affects the cardiovascular system, it should not be discontinued abruptly, but rather slowly over several days. Abrupt withdrawal in patients with coronary heart disease may aggravate coronary problems and lead to unstable angina or myocardial infarction (heart attack).

Other Beta Blockers

If propranolol is not recommended, treatment with another beta blocker may be considered. Timolol, commonly known as Blocadren, has also received approval for migraine prevention. Both timolol and nadolol, commonly known as Corzide, have demonstrated successful migraine prevention in many patients. For asthmatics or those with bronchial disorders, a "cardioselective" beta blocker, such as metoprolol (marketed as Lopressor or Toprol) or atenolol (commonly known as Tenormin) may be substituted.

Divalproex Sodium

Divalproex sodium, commonly known as Depakote, is the most recent agent approved for migraine prevention. It has been used as an anticonvulsant since 1983, and has also been used effectively for some psychiatric conditions. Its success in preventing migraine may be due to its capacity to increase levels of the amino acid GABA, which is believed to be a player in migraine development. Divalproex sodium can be considered first-line therapy for patients with coexisting seizures, mania, or anxiety. Its side effects include nausea, gastrointestinal distress, sedation, tremor, pancreatitis, some blood disorders, and liver toxicity. Complete blood counts and liver function tests should be obtained prior to therapy and at frequent intervals thereafter, especially during the first six months of treatment. This drug can be considered safe for prolonged treatment.

Methysergide

Methysergide, commonly known as Sansert, is a synthetic drug that is closely related to the naturally occurring ergotamine medications. Although methysergide is one of the most effective agents for migraine prevention, it generally is reserved for use in patients with frequent, severe, disabling migraines that do not respond to less-toxic agents. The adverse effects associated with this agent include nausea, vomiting, abdominal pain, insomnia, drowsiness, leg cramps, numbness, fluid retention, weight gain, hair loss, and low blood pressure. Long-term use of methysergide has been associated with production of fibrous tissues of the lining of the kidney and lungs, and fibrotic thickening of the cardiac valves. Therefore, patients on methysergide therapy should be evaluated at regular intervals to make sure that the fibrous tissue has not developed. Patients cannot be kept on therapy with methysergide for more than four to six months consecutively, and should be given a four- to six-week drug-free interval between treatment periods. The drug is not recommended in patients with a history of collagen diseases or fibrotic disorders, as well as peripheral vascular disease, coronary artery disease, severe hypertension, and thrombophlebitis.

Calcium Channel Blockers

The effectiveness of the calcium channel blockers in migraine prevention appears to be related to their ability to inhibit spasm in the arteries, as well as to block platelet serotonin release and platelet clumping. Their full effects may not be realized for two to four weeks after initiation of treatment. Although these agents have been studied extensively in Europe and the United States for migraine prevention, no calcium channel blocker has received approval for migraine prevention. In the United States, these drugs are used to treat hypertension and certain heart problems.

Verapamil (marketed as Calan, Isoptin, or Verelan) is a calcium-entry blocker. The drug maintains its effects, which promotes its usefulness as a migraine preventive agent. Constipation is among the most common side effects of therapy, but, as with any of the calcium blockers, flushing, light-headedness, hypotension, rash, and nausea may also occur.

Nimodipine, commonly known as Nimotop, has been effective in preventing migraine, but it has also been associated with more behavioral changes, sedation, and other central nervous system (CNS) effects than other calcium blockers. Muscle pains have also been reported.

Patients using calcium channel blockers should be monitored carefully for adverse symptoms related to postural hypotension (low blood pressure associated with changing position). This is especially important in patients who are also taking other antihypertensive agents, such as the beta blockers. Calcium channel blockers should be used with caution in patients with concomitant congestive heart failure. Abrupt withdrawal of these agents should be avoided because of their potential to induce chest pain, rebound angina, or exacerbation of symptoms.

Antidepressants

The antimigraine effect of the antidepressant agents is believed to be relatively independent of their antidepressant effect, although the exact relationship remains uncertain. Tricyclic antidepressants (TCAs) are known to block the reabsorption of serotonin. There is a two- to three-week lag time that generally occurs between initiation of treatment and the appearance of therapeutic effects.

TCAs are not considered to be first choice in migraine preventive therapy, but may be useful in some patients, particularly those with coexisting migraine and tension-type headache. Amitriptyline, commonly known as Elavil, is one of the oldest antidepressants used in migraine therapy, along with doxepin (commonly known as Sinequan), nortriptyline, and imipramine. These antidepressants tend to be more sedating than protriptyline (commonly known as Vivactil) or desipramine, commonly known as Norpramin. These agents may also cause constipation, dry mouth, weight gain, blurred vision, rapid heart beat, hypotension, sexual dysfunction, and urinary retention, and are not recommended in patients with narrow-angle glaucoma, prostate problems, or cardiac conduction disturbances.

Some of the newer antidepressants, including the serotonin reuptake inhibitors (SSRIs) and others, appear to operate more specifically at serotonin receptors—a more targeted attack—and have different side effects that are less disabling. As with the TCAs, however, a lag time of two to three weeks may occur before therapeutic effects are evident. Among the serotonin reuptake inhibitors, fluoxetine (well known as Prozac), sertraline (commonly known as Zoloft), and paroxetine (commonly known as Paxil) have been beneficial. However, nausea, insomnia, agitation, weight loss, and sexual dysfunction may be associated with their use. Among the other antidepressants, bupropion (commonly known as Wellbutrin) and trazodone (commonly known as Desyrel) have demonstrated some efficacy in migraine prevention. Bupropion, however, has been known to produce agitation, anxiety, insomnia, and seizures, and is therefore not recommended for use in patients with a history of seizures, or those who are prone to eating disorders (e.g., bulimics). Trazodone has been associated with priapism (persistent erection of the penis with pain and tenderness) and should be avoided in male migraineurs.

Of the monoamine oxidase inhibitors (MAOIs), phenelzine (commonly known as Nardil) and isocarboxazid (commonly known as Marplan) have been found to be helpful in the preventative treatment of migraine. Mono-amine oxidase (MAO) has been identified as one of the chemicals instrumental in migraine development, and these drugs prevent some of its actions. These agents are not first-line antidepressant therapy, but may be considered for use when other treatments fail. Drugs that inhibit MAO activity have a wide range of clinical effects and must be monitored with extreme caution due to their potential interaction with several foods and drugs.

Adverse effects reported with MAOIs include dizziness, insomnia, hypomania, orthostatic hypotension, dry mouth, blurred vision, urinary retention, impotence, edema in the feet, ankles, and hands, as well as weight gain. Patients should be warned to avoid alcoholic beverages, tyramine-containing foods, and certain drugs. When the body's MAO is inhibited, ingestion of large amounts of tyramine may result in serious high blood pressure of sufficient severity to cause heart attack or a stroke. Due to the residual MAOI effects, a two-week "wash out" period is necessary before tyramine-containing foods or interactive drugs may be ingested.

Clonidine

Clonidine (commonly known as Catapres) is a centrally acting alpha blocker that acts on the part of the brain that subsequently affects the blood vessels. Its efficacy in migraine prevention is not comparable to the beta blockers. Clonidine has been found to be particularly helpful, however, in those patients who experience food-related attacks. It is also effective in those patients withdrawing from opiates (narcotics). Side effects associated with clonidine include drowsiness, dry mouth, constipation, disturbances of ejaculation, orthostatic hypertension, and depression.

Cyproheptadine

Cyproheptadine has been used successfully in the treatment of childhood migraine. Its anti-serotonin and anti-histamine effects have suggested its use for treatment of migraine in adults, although results in this category have been marginal. Sedation and excessive weight gain also limit its usefulness.

NSAIDs

The NSAIDs have a unique place in the treatment of migraine, in that their anti-inflammatory and analgesic properties make them appropriate choices for abortive, symptomatic, and prophylactic therapy. The NSAIDs are platelet antagonists and prevent platelet clumping—an action associated with migraine development. They also affect the levels of serotonin. NSAIDs are of particular interest in the preventative treatment of those who suffer from chronic migraine. Data collected from the U.S. Physicians' Health Study suggest the possibility that regular use of aspirin or other platelet-active drugs in this category might reduce the recurrence of migraine by approximately 20 percent.

Gastrointestinal complaints are the adverse side effects most often reported with this category of drugs. The risk of GI complaints escalates with increased dose (thus, the lowest possible dose should be used), chronic use, alcohol ingestion, smoking, and in patients with a history of peptic ulcer disease. Patients should be monitored for GI bleeding, and for evidence of liver and/or kidney disease, both of which have been associated with chronic NSAID use.

Preventive Techniques for Specific Types of Migraine

Prolonged Migraine

Occasionally, a migraine attack lasts over twenty-four hours. It is believed that in this situation, a sterile inflammation (one that is not caused by an infection) is surrounding the widened blood vessel responsible for the migraine attack. Corticosteroids are given to the patient to decrease this inflammation and hasten the end of the prolonged migraine. The corticosteroid may be given as an injection or orally over several days.

Coexisting Migraine and Tension-Type Headaches

The use of antidepressants is especially helpful in coexisting migraine with tension-type headaches and migraine patients with associated depression. Because of the complex nature of these headaches, combination therapy may be indicated. Combined therapy may involve a tricyclic antidepressant and an MAOI. Previously combined therapy with these two classes of drugs was not recommended. Prescribing this combination therapy should only be undertaken by a physician familiar with the actions of both agents. I recommend that combination therapy should be started only in a specialized inpatient headache unit, where appropriate monitoring is possible. Combination therapy should be limited to patients who have been unresponsive to conventional therapy.

In order to prevent both types of headache, the therapy may involve an antidepressant and a beta blocker, such as propranolol, or the calcium channel blockers. The NSAIDs have also been effective in treating coexisting migraine and tension-type headaches.

Hormonal Headaches

• *Menstrual migraine*

In the preventive and abortive therapy of menstrual migraine, the medications of choice are the nonsteroidal anti-inflammatory agents (NSAIDs). As a rule, treatment should be initiated starting two to three days before the onset of the period and continued through the flow. Because the treatment interval is brief, there is limited risk of gastrointestinal adverse effects. The NSAIDs used most frequently include: fenoprofen calcium (commonly known as Nalfon), ketoprofen, ketorolac, nabumetone (commonly known as Relafen), naproxen (commonly known as Naprosyn), and naproxen sodium. Another NSAID can be considered if the first type is ineffective. For those patients who do not respond to NSAID therapy, small doses of ergotamine agents may be considered for preventive treatment without risk of developing ergot dependence. Ergotamine tartrate may be prescribed at bedtime or twice daily. A combination agent, containing ergotamine tartrate, phenobarbital, and belladonna alkaloids (commonly known as Bellergal-S), may be given two or three times a day, starting three days before and continuing through the menstrual flow.

Alternative agents include methylergonovine maleate (commonly known as Methergine), and dihydroergotamine (DHE) may be quite effective in preventing or terminating severe menstrual migraine (see chapter 9).

Methysergide may also be considered for short-term therapy. The risks usually associated with methysergide therapy, such as kidney, lung, or cardiac fibrosis, are decreased due to the brief treatment interval. The triptans (chapter 9) have also been used on a daily basis for prevention during times the patient is at risk. Preventive therapy can also involve the use of other agents at period time—such as the beta blockers. Other migraine preventive drugs, such as divalproex sodium, calcium channel blockers, antidepressants, or alpha agonists, may be considered for the patient with menstrual migraine. When the patient is already on migraine preventive therapy, the dose may be increased prior to menses.

For the abortive therapy, those agents used in nonmenstrual migraine are indicated. The triptans such as sumatriptan, naratriptan, rizatriptan, and zolmitriptan are effective in migraine abortive therapy. Other abortive agents include DHE, ergotamine tartrate, isometheptene mucate, and a combination agent of aspirin, acetaminophen, and caffeine. These drugs have been described previously in chapter 9.

Hormonal therapy used to treat menstrual migraine can include estrogens, estrogen antagonists, estrogens in combination with testosterone or progesterone, and prolactin-release inhibitors. These agents are used to prevent an increase in estrogen during the luteal phase of the menstrual cycle and/or its subsequent drop. Other successful therapies include replacement of estrogen prior to the period. Establishing stable estrogen levels can be attained via estradiol gel, estradiol skin patches, or at least one estradiol implant. In some individuals with intractable menstrual migraine, particularly if severe pain with menses is also present, oral contraceptive use may be effective in prophylaxis of menstrual migraine, as the birth control pills stabilize the levels of estrogen.

- *PMS headaches*

  For the treatment of headaches that occur during the premenstrual phase, aspirin and other NSAIDs can be effective. Acetaminophen is not used because it has no anti-inflammatory properties. Therapy to stop ovulation, such as the oral contraceptives, may be considered in severe cases.

- *Pregnancy*

  The gold standard of treatment during pregnancy is no treatment. For example, ergotamines and other vasoconstrictors cause changes in the uterus and should not be used during pregnancy. However, sporadic use of sumatriptan may be considered a safe option during pregnancy. For those patients experiencing migraine during pregnancy, acetaminophen may be considered for pain relief. After the first trimester, caffeine, most of the NSAIDs, butorphanol, and narcotics are relatively safe in providing analgesia. Prophylactic treatment may be instituted after the first trimester, and the drugs include tricyclic antidepressants, fluoxetine, or propranolol.

  It is important that you talk to your obstetrician during

your pregnancy about headache treatment. If you are also under the care of a headache specialist, a consultation between the physicians is essential.

- *Breast-feeding*

For prophylactic treatment during lactation (breast-feeding), the agents considered safe include the beta blockers, calcium channel blockers, fluoxetine (commonly known as Prozac), and sertraline (marketed as Zoloft). For those breast-feeding patients who require abortive therapy, sumatriptan can be used, but it will be necessary to use the breast pump for four hours after using the drug, and then dispose of the milk.

- *Menopause*

The current popularity of hormone-replacement therapy (HRT) is not limited to its relief of menopausal symptoms but includes prevention of heart disease and osteoporosis. In individuals with a prior history of migraine, the lowest possible dose of estrogen should be used on an uninterrupted basis and not cyclic dosing—on twenty-one days, off seven days. This procedure maintains a stable level of estrogen. If you should encounter any problems, another form of estrogen can be utilized. The estradiol skin patch appears beneficial in maintaining plasma estrogen levels. You should be proactive in the decision-making process about HRT. Administration of low-dose estrogen, occasionally combined with testosterone, may be effective for those women not using HRT but who experience persistent or recent onset migraine attacks at menopause.

• *Headaches associated with oral contraceptive use*
Despite the potential for migraine headaches posed by oral contraceptives, many women continue to take the Pill. If you are reluctant to discontinue the oral contraceptive, an NSAID, starting on the twentieth day of the cycle and continued until the second day of the next cycle, may be effective in preventing or decreasing the severity of migraine attacks that occur during the week off the oral contraceptives. A newer low-dose oral contraceptive on a noncycling basis (on twenty-eight days of the month without a break), used for three to six months, may be an effective alternative. Estradiol skin patches may also be used during the seven-day interval when you are not taking the active drug.

Childhood Migraine

Certain factors influence the treatment of children with migraine:

• Age of the patient
• Size of the patient
• Frequency of the headaches
• Severity of the headaches

Elimination diets, avoidance of usual headache triggers, and biofeedback are all utilized in the treatment of the child with migraine. If the child is experiencing frequent headaches, a preventive agent may be considered—such as cyproheptadine and propranolol. Children should not be treated with addicting agents, such as the narcotics and barbiturates. Children will usually find relief from the attack by sleeping, along with mild over-the-counter pain reliever.

Case Report

Since sophomore year in high school, Vince Bailey always seemed to be the center of attention—especially during football season. When I first saw Vince at the clinic, he was a junior at a Big Ten university, probably bound for the Rose Bowl in January, and in the hunt for the Heisman Trophy. It was difficult to imagine that this strong, healthy, and robust twenty-year-old running back was suffering from any malady, particularly migraines.

When Vince was in junior high, he did experience an occasional severe headache—similar to the attacks his mother suffered. The headaches did not force him to miss school or any athletic competition. His parents noticed that Vince often complained of headaches after a celebration—meaning a party with pizza, and quite often chocolate ice cream. Those items were two of Vince's favorites.

At that time, his mother wisely stopped these treats and the headaches seemed to be under control.

Vince's football career in high school had been phenomenal. The varsity teams made their way to the state finals three times—and during his senior year, they became state champions. Vince was all-state in football, honorable mention in basketball, and was acknowledged as a formidable pitcher on the school's baseball team. He also was an excellent student and no one was surprised when he was recruited by several colleges with well-known football traditions. In his first two years of college, he was even mentioned in several national sports magazines.

And now everything seemed to be coming together for Vince and the university. They were ranked in the top ten preseason, and were expected to win the Big Ten championship and a trip to Pasadena. Everything was coming up roses—that is, until the team flew to West Virginia for a nonconference game, early in September. The migraine attack hit Vince early on game day. He couldn't focus his eyes, and he was vomiting. The team physician was concerned, and took a brief headache history. Yes, Vince had headaches when he was younger—but they were related to food triggers. And, yes, Vince's mother had migraine headaches. The physician quickly diagnosed migraine, and ordered a triptan—Imitrex—in the hopes that the headache would be relieved. As quickly as the headache started, it seemed to diminish. Vince was ready to play by the second quarter, and he ran for over seventy yards. It was a great victory—and a great day for Vince.

The coaches and Vince were concerned that he might again by sidelined by a headache. An appointment was made at our clinic, and I concurred with the team physician—Vince was suffering from migraine without aura. Preventive therapy was not indicated, but I would also use a triptan at the first signs of a migraine attack. For the next few weeks, Vince was doing well—no headaches. But during the second week of November, the team had one week's hiatus—and Vince's sister was getting married. He flew home on Friday, and by Saturday morning, he had a terrible headache. The triptan helped, but the headache recurred on Sunday, and he and his parents were concerned.

On Monday, Vince asked for an emergency appointment. What could he do if each time he was on a plane, he got a headache? After all, Pasadena seemed his destiny on New Year's Day, and he would have to fly out to California. I reassured Vince that many migraine patients are prone to headaches when they change altitudes. I would prescribe a diuretic, acetazolamide (commonly known as Diamox), to take starting two days prior to the plane trip. We could test my theory when he flew to New York City for the Heisman presentation. It worked—no headache (unfortunately, no Heisman either). I reassured Vince that I thought the trip to the Rose Bowl would be uneventful (for headaches), and since he was a junior, he could be eligible for next year's Heisman. If a headache should appear, the triptan had been effective in the past—and he would have a few days between arriving in California and the big game.

Again, no headache, but Vince did come home with the Rose Bowl Trophy. The team physician phoned me to say there had been no other incidence of headaches since November, and it looked as if Vince was going pro after this year. I hope he remembered to fill his prescription when the next away game occurred!

CHAPTER 11
Alternative Medicine and Migraine

Ulysses S. Grant (1822–1885), who served as eighteenth president of the United States, experienced one of his well-known migraine attacks on the evening of April 8, 1865, during the Civil War. From Grant's journal entry for that date, we learn of his unconventional treatment for an acute migraine:

I was suffering very severely with a sick headache, and stopped at a farm house on the road some distance to the rear of the main body of the army. I spent the night in bathing my feet in hot water and mustard, and putting mustard plasters on my wrists and the back part of my neck, hoping to be cured by morning.

Unfortunately, the headache remained when the general awakened. Soon after he arose, a messenger arrived with a communication from General Lee, who was willing to talk peace terms. Grant's next journal entry reports:

When the officer reached me, I was still suffering from the sick headache; but the instant I saw the contents of the note I was cured.

Was it the mustard plaster or the Confederate general's capitulation? For many headache sufferers, they would give credit to the plaster. Alternative therapies have become increasingly popular with the consumer. What alternative treatment options does the migraine sufferer have?

Unconventional therapy has been used for many chronic conditions, including back pain, allergies, arthritis, and headache. In a recent survey, 13 percent of the respondents reported a headache as a complaint, for which 27 percent had used unconventional therapy in the previous twelve months. Relaxation techniques and chiropractic treatment were the most commonly used nondrug therapies. In a 1990 survey, it was estimated that 34 percent of Americans had used at least one alternative therapy in the prior year. One-third had consulted an alternative provider on average of nineteen times per year. The most frequent consumers of alternative therapy were whites, aged twenty-five to forty-nine years, who were better educated and in the upper income group. Most of these consumers did not tell their physicians about their visits to alternative medicine providers. Usually, they were seeking relief from chronic, non-life-threatening conditions (back pain, arthritis, headache, insomnia).

In 1990, approximately $13.7 billion was used for alternative therapies, of which $10.3 billion was not covered by third party carriers. The federal government has established an Office of Alternative Medicine, which provided thirty grants of $30,000 each. Most of these grants were for treatments that some, including myself, would consider "quack" therapies, including the following: (1) acupuncture for depression; (2) massage therapy for HIV-related conditions; (3) music therapy for psychosocial adjustment post–brain injury; (4) hypnosis for accelerated fracture healing; (5) classical homeopathy's impact on health status (homeopathy was developed by the German physician Samuel Hahnemann, who believed that the ability of a substance to cure a disease emerges from its power to cause symptoms in a healthy person that are similar to those of the disease itself. This is known as the "Law of Similars"); (6) guided imagery for asthma; and (7) prayer intervention for substance abuse.

Case Report

Phil McNulty is a sixty-four-year-old accountant, who has been a longtime patient at the clinic. He first saw me twenty-five years ago and was diagnosed with migraine without aura. Over the years, he has developed a depressive component to the headaches, usually associated with stress at work. He has been treated successfully with the calcium channel blockers and antidepressants (see chapter 10). For his acute headaches, he uses the isometheptene mucate combination, commonly known as Midrin (chapter 9), and occasionally an NSAID. His headaches were very manageable and he would only consult with me every four to six months.

On a spring visit, Phil complained of an increase in headache frequency. But of course he said, it was probably related to "April fifteenth pressure." A neurological exam on that date was negative, and we discussed ordering a CT scan. When he first came to see me in 1976, CT scans were not commonly in use and the skull X rays that were performed on Phil were negative. On this most recent visit, Phil agreed to have a CT scan. The scan was negative, and now I had to wonder why Phil's headaches had increased. I asked him to come back in six weeks, and we would see if there was any further change in the headaches.

At the next visit, in early summer, Phil told me that the headaches were coming one to three times per week, and the attacks were harder to manage. He was using more Midrin, and was also using an over-the-counter pain reliever, usually ibuprofen or naproxen sodium. I asked him if he had gotten any other prescription drugs from his internist—possibly he was taking a nitrate medication, which can exacerbate headaches. No, he hadn't started anything new, but his wife was using herbal remedies and had encouraged him to use *Ginkgo biloba* to help his memory and overall health in general. Phil said he hadn't noticed any change in his memory—or well-being. I suggested that he stop the herbal therapy for four weeks and see if he noted any improvement in the headaches. One month later, Phil called and said he thought he could reasonably delay his appointment. After stopping the herbal agents, he had only one headache. I told him how happy I was that he was again managing his headaches. However, I couldn't do anything for his memory! I concluded from this incident that herbal remedies may be beneficial but, for the patient with migraine, caution must be used. Your innate sensitivities make you prone to headache with any type of change. When in doubt, discuss the use of any medication or alternative form of therapy with your physician.

Herbal Remedies

Feverfew

One specific herb used for headache is feverfew, and it has been used as a folk remedy for migraine for many years. Studies have been conducted on migraine sufferers who ate fresh leaves of the feverfew plant in sandwiches, crushed with honey, or as icing on sugar pills. Seventy percent of these subjects claimed that their migraine attacks were less frequent or less severe, and 33 percent claimed that the migraine attacks were resolved. Thirty percent reported no benefit from this remedy. However, the studies were not adequately controlled, and other researchers have not been able to duplicate the results. Side effects have been reported with feverfew, including skin rash and sore mouth. Feverfew works like the NSAIDs in relieving inflammation. However, the NSAIDs appear to be more effective in aborting migraine attacks, as well as relieving migraine pain.

Saint-John's-wort

Saint-John's-wort is the common name for the flowering plant *Hypericum perforatum,* and has been recommended for the treatment of depression. This herb has many active ingredients, including hypericum extract, which inhibits uptake of serotonin, norepinephrine, and dopamine. It has been reported that Saint-John's-wort is effective for mild and moderate depression, and is generally tolerable. But if the studies are reviewed, the diagnosis of depression has not been firmly established. Various doses were used, and trials on these agents were limited.

If you suffer from major depression, especially with concomitant migraine, you should have an extensive medical workup, and possibly psychiatric evaluation. Unfortunately, using herbal therapy along with prescription medications could produce serious side effects.

Herb-Drug Interactions

The following is a list of frequently used herbs and the drugs (usually used for headaches) with which they inter-act and produce serious symptoms:

Herb	Prescription Agent	Side Effect
• Saint-John's-wort	Paroxetine (Paxil)	Lethargy/incoherence
(Hypericum	Trazodone (Desyrel)	Mild serotonergic symptoms
perforatum)	Sertraline (Zoloft)	Mild serotonergic symptoms
—used for	Nefazodone (Serzone)	Mild serotonergic symptoms
depression, memory	Some oral contraceptives	Breakthrough menstrual bleeding
• Ginkgo *(Ginkgo*	Aspirin	Spontaneous bleeding
biloba)	Ergotamine with caffeine	Bleeding in the brain
—believed to help	(Wigraine, Ercaf)	
increase blood flow to	Phenelzine (Nardil)	Headache, tremor, mania
the brain, and help	Lithium	Decreased concentration
memory		

Vitamins/Minerals

Riboflavin (Vitamin B$_2$)

There have been reports that large doses of vitamin B$_2$ have helped improve migraine headaches. The number of subjects in the study were small, and larger studies would be needed to confirm the usefulness of this treatment. The only side effect reported with this treatment was diarrhea. Vitamin B_2 is found in beans, cheese, eggs, fish, meat, poultry, spinach, and yogurt.

Magnesium

It is well known that a deficiency in magnesium causes narrowing of the blood vessels. This effect on the blood vessels has prompted researchers to investigate the role of magnesium in the development of migraine and they have concluded that maintaining adequate amounts of magnesium in your diet may help prevent migraine attacks. At recommended daily allowances, magnesium does not cause side effects. But if the recommended doses are exceeded, the patient may experience drowsiness, weakness, and lethargy. Patients with kidney disorders and the elderly are especially vulnerable to toxic effects, which can be lethal.

Magnesium is found in wheat bran, whole grains, dark green leafy vegetables (spinach), meat, nuts, beans, milk, and bananas. Again, the migraine sufferer may find some help in following a diet that includes these items.

Marijuana

Research continues into the pharmacological properties of cannabis and related substances. In one study, migraine attacks occurred in three patients after the abrupt discontinuation of long-term marijuana use—attributed to changes in vasoconstriction (narrowing of the blood vessels) and the antiplatelet effects (causing the platelets to clump and adhere to the walls of the blood vessels) of the substances in marijuana (cannabinoids).

Air Ionization

Many migraine sufferers will identify changes in weather and/or altitude as headache triggers. Various hot, dry winds, such as the

- Santa Ana winds of California
- Desert winds of Arizona
- Chinook in Canada
- Sirocco of Italy
- Föhn of the European Alps
- Mistral of France

have also been linked to migraine headaches—due to an increase in the number of small ionized particles in the air, with the greater proportion of these particles positively charged and affecting barometric pressure. Because of these environmental triggers, there has been development of small electrical devices that deliver negative ions into a room. The biological effects of charged ions are not well understood, and the use of air ionization machines for migraine prevention is debatable.

Acupuncture

Acupuncture, originating in China, has become popular in the Western world. It is used for a variety of ailments, including migraine. It involves the use of puncture with long needles, according to the ancient Asian system, and patients with identifiable tender spots on the head and neck are more likely to respond to acupuncture. But research into the use of acupuncture versus conventional therapy of migraine has been inconclusive. Although it may not be beneficial as a single treatment, it might help relieve pain if used in addition to traditional drug therapy.

At our clinic, we use sterile, disposable needles that are inserted into various points on the body which, according to acupuncture tradition, trigger headache.

My interest in acupuncture started with Richard Nixon's first trip to China in 1972. The *New York Times* reporter John Reston needed an appendectomy while accompanying the president on this diplomatic trip. During the surgery, acupuncture was used instead of anesthetic drugs. Because of Reston's saga, the press highlighted this ancient Chinese practice, and the general public as well as health practitioners were keenly interested in this alternative therapy. Dealing with headache patients on a daily basis, I too was interested in learning this technique as a possible remedy for my patients. My recourse was to travel to London for an intense training course under the tutelage of Dr. Felix Mann, a renowned acupuncturist who had written extensively on the subject. On my return, I began to use acupuncture on a few select cases—with some success. However, I found that acupuncture was beneficial as an adjunct to other, more conventional, forms of therapy. It was not a substitute for these other treatment modalities.

The Chinese have long held that the individual has vital pain control points along various meridians of the body. Meridians are areas of the body surface that are thought to control various functions of the body. By blocking these meridians, via acupuncture, pain such as headache may be relieved. Others believe that acupuncture positively influences a balance between mind and body. On a positive note, there are no significant adverse effects from acupuncture—a factor which is a comfort to many patients.

Hydrotherapy

The use of hydrotherapy, alternating hot and cold compresses or showers as a method of treating headaches, including migraine, is recommended by some physical therapists and some older physicians. Although we use the application of cold to the site of the headache (via ice bag or cold pack), we do not encourage hydrotherapy for patients at the Diamond Headache Clinic.

Transcutaneous Electrical Stimulation

Electrotherapy was first suggested by Guillaume-Benjamin-Amand Duchenne (1806–1875), a French neurologist, who was the first to describe several nervous and muscular disorders. The use of transcutaneous electrical nerve stimulators (TENS) for chronic pain can trace their origins with this form of therapy.

During the past three decades, many types of chronic pain have been treated with both spinal cord electrical stimulation and TENS. TENS involves the production and transmission of electrical energy from the surface of the skin to the nervous system. The rationale for this therapy is the process by which the small, uncovered pain fibers can be controlled by the larger, covered fibers—thus reducing pain. The control of these fibers will manage pain symptoms. The efficacy of TENS has been demonstrated in conditions such as phantom pain, chronic back disorders, and headache. For headaches, the TENS instrument—a small stimulator—is connected to electrodes placed on the skin's surface, usually over the site of the pain. The patient can control the amount of stimulation for a specified interval, about five to ten minutes. The results seen at our clinic have been marginal.

Other Medical Disciplines

Homeopathy

Homeopathic medicine was introduced by Samuel Hahnemann in Philadelphia, which remains the site of a medical school named for this early American physician. At one time, this medical discipline was practiced by many physicians throughout the United States and Europe.

As we discussed earlier, the "Law of Similars" is the basis for the theory of Hahnemann's "likes cures." This theory illustrated the ability of a substance to cure a disease based on its power to cause symptoms in a healthy person which are similar to the disease itself. That is, by using agents which produce a similar effect to the symptoms of a particular disease, the body's resistance to this disease is increased.

Consumers can still find many homeopathic preparations sold over-the-counter in health food stores. However, the number of physicians who continue to use this form of medicine has greatly diminished.

Chiropractic Medicine

Who are the chiropractors and what do they do for patients with headaches and other forms of chronic pain? There are two subdivisions of chiropractic medicine. One type believes that manual manipulation of the spinal column and nerves is effective in treating various conditions. The other division uses physical manipulation of the spine combined with other treatments, including nutritional consultation.

In treating headache, these practitioners focus on the muscles and bones as they believe that headaches—whether migraine or tension-type—emerge from the bone and muscles, as well as the blood and nerves. By using physical manipulation, they believe that they can alter bodily functions and disorders. This physical manipulation—commonly known as adjustments—is believed to relieve whatever is causing the headache.

I would caution headache patients who are considering chiropractic treatment to consult a physician to evaluate their headache condition, and rule out any possible organic disorders via laboratory and radiologic tests. There is a potential risk from manipulation of the spine, especially the neck, with some dire consequences.

CHAPTER 12
Resources for Help and Education

Educating migraine sufferers and their families is an essential in preventing headaches. In addition to instruction provided by the health care team, you may require or desire further information.

Part of an initial visit at a specialized headache clinic is directed at educating you about the diagnosis of the headaches, as well as options for treatment. The health care team will review the various migraine triggers, and provide a calendar for you to maintain to help identify migraine precipitants. You will probably receive an elimination diet, listing the foods that are recognized as possible migraine triggers. Instructions on lifestyle will also be provided—to insure that you maintain a sleep and meal schedule to help avoid further incidents of migraine attacks. The nuances of headache therapy will also be reviewed, and must be individualized for you.

If you are admitted to an inpatient headache unit, a variety of educational programs are provided by the multidisciplinary health care team. You will be encouraged to attend classes with a staff pharmacist and dietitian. Also, art therapy and leisure activity classes may be held. Other classes include relaxation exercises, stress management, and coping skills. The goal of these programs is to aid you in using self-help techniques to prevent headaches and decrease the severity of the migraine attacks.

Physician organizations can also offer information to headache sufferers and their families. The American Headache Society (formerly known as the American Association for the Study of Headache) was founded in 1959 for physicians and other health care practitioners interested in headache management.

Their address is: **The American Headache Society, 19 Mantua Road, Mount Royal, NJ 08061, (609) 423-0043. For referrals: (609) 845-0322, fax: (609) 423-0082, www.aash.org.**

There are several professional journals that are dedicated to topics concerning headache treatment and research. The official journal of the American Headache Society is *Headache,* and the official journal of the International Headache Society is titled *Cephalalgia.* I serve as editor-in-chief of *Headache Quarterly: Current Treatment and Research,* which is supported by the Diamond Headache Clinic Research and Educational Foundation. All of these organizations sponsor postgraduate courses for physicians and other health practitioners interested in headache management.

For those individuals seeking information on headaches and treatment, the National Headache Foundation serves as a resource organization, disseminating information. The foundation also sponsors seminars throughout the country in which physicians interested in headache management lecture about various types of headache. It also sponsors research into the causes and treatments of headache by providing grants to researchers in the field. The foundation will provide a list of physicians in your local area who are members of the foundation and who are interested in headache management, as well as support groups in your community.

The foundation is located at: **The National Headache Foundation, 423 West St. James Place, 2nd Floor, Chicago, IL 60614-2750, (800) 843-2256, fax: (773) 525-7357, www.headaches.org.**

There is a plethora of information available on the World Wide Web. A major source of information on all things headache is the World Headache Alliance (WHA)—a global alliance of lay organizations whose aim is to provide a comprehensive, and frequently updated, information service for headache sufferers, as well as their families and friends. The official Web site of the WHA is WHAT! (World Headache Alliance Telelink). The purpose of WHAT! is to facilitate communication between fellow headache sufferers, their physicians, and their local patient-based WHA member organizations. The Web site at www.w-h-a.org/what is also used to direct sufferers to what the WHA believes to be the most helpful resources and information sources on headache disorders available on the Internet today. The Web site also has information on professional journals and books for the headache sufferer and physicians interested in headache management.

Headache and migraine sites that may be of interest to you, the headache sufferer, include the following:

- National Headache Foundation: www.headaches.org
- Migraine Sufferers Support Group: www.migraine.co.nz
- ACHE (American Council on Headache Education): www.achenet.org
- International Headache Society: www.i-h-s.org
- ALADEC (LinkLand Espanol)

To reach the home page of the Migraine Association of Canada, the Internet address is www.migraine.ca. Similar to the National Headache Foundation, the Migraine Association of Canada is dedicated to:

- Being Canada's source of education and information on migraine and its medical, social, and economic effects;
- Creating public awareness of the serious nature of migraine;
- Fostering a greater understanding of, and compassion for, migraine sufferers;
- Supporting research for a cure.

This association publishes a newsletter *(Headlines)*, and has produced two booklets—*Migraine Friendly Cookbook* and *Managing Migraine in the Workplace.*

A multitude of books have been published on the subject of headaches. It is important for you to know that you are not alone, and that help is available. These books include:

- *Taking Control of Your Headaches: How to Get the Treatment You Need,* updated version, by P. N. Duckro, W. D. Richardson, and J. E. Marshall. New York: Guildford Press, 1999.
- *The Headache Alternative,* by A. Mauskop, and M. A. Brill. New York: Dell Publishing, 1997.
- *The Hormone Headache,* by S. Diamond, B. Still, and C. Still. New York: Macmillan, 1995.
- *Headache and Diet: Tyramine-Free Recipes,* by S. Diamond, D. Francis, A. Diamond Vye. Madison, Connecticut: International Universities Press, 1993.

GLOSSARY

Acupuncture. Acupuncture is an ancient Chinese remedy for a variety of illnesses. It is based on the theory that by stimulating nerves, one can block pain. The puncture acts as a counterirritant to stop the painful impulses from radiating up the spinal cord. Some patients have responded to the use of acupuncture in headache treatment in conjunction with traditional methods of therapy.

Alpha Agonists. These drugs, which have shown some effectiveness in migraine, were originally used in the treatment of hypertension. The most commonly used alpha agonist, clonidine, has shown marginal success in migraine therapy, except for those patients with a particular sensitivity to tyramine-containing foods.

Antidepressants. As their name suggests, these medications are used for depression. For patients with chronic headache, these drugs are useful for their mood-elevating properties as well as their analgesic actions. The drugs are especially helpful for those headache patients with a sleep disturbance.

Anxiety Headache. This is a form of chronic tension-type headache that is related to an underlying anxiety. The anxiety may be indicated by job complaints or stress. The patient may complain of a sleep disturbance in the form of difficulty falling asleep.

Arteriography. A method to see the blood vessels by injecting a dye or inserting a catheter.

Aura. The aura of migraine consists of neurological signs of an impending headache. Usually the aura refers to a variety of visual symptoms, including seeing bright or flashing lights, zigzag lines, distorted size, shape, and location, and even losing part of the visual field. Patients also may experience hallucinations in hearing and smell prior to the onset of the migraine attack. Other patients may notice numbness or tingling in their arms or legs before the migraine headache starts.

Beta Blockers. These drugs act by blocking the action of certain substances, such as adrenaline, found in the body. Previously used in the treatment of hypertension and cardiac problems, these drugs have demonstrated their effectiveness in preventing migraine. The only beta blockers approved for migraine treatment are propranolol and timolol. Patients with respiratory problems may not be able to tolerate those beta blockers, which are not selective, and should be started on a cardio-selective beta blocker, such as metoprolol.

Biofeedback. Biofeedback is a technique that trains the patient to control a previously unused or involuntarily controlled function of the body, such as heart rate, blood pressure, muscle tension, and temperature. It is used in a variety of medical conditions and is particularly effective with migraine and tension headaches. The control is achieved through training with a monitor that measures these bodily functions. The monitor feeds back information about the bodily function to the patient, and through various methods (diaphragmatic breathing, relaxation phases), the patient learns to control that particular function. Biofeedback also uses self-hypnotic techniques or progressive relaxation.

Caffeine. Caffeine is commonly known as an ingredient in coffee, tea, and cola beverages. It is also a frequent ingredient in over-the-counter analgesics. In some preparations of ergotamine, caffeine is added to potentiate the absorption of the ergotamine. Unfortunately, many patients overconsume caffeine, whether in beverages or over-the-counter analgesics. When the source of caffeine is skipped, the patient will experience a caffeine-withdrawal headache. These headaches most often occur when someone is fasting or on weekends when the person delays or skips a morning cup of coffee.

Calcium Channel Blockers. Calcium channel blockers are used for heart disease and for patients recovering from stroke. These drugs act by stabilizing the cranial blood vessels. By maintaining a balance in these blood vessels, they also prevent the brain from being exposed to an oxygen deficiency. Expansion of the blood vessels is acknowledged as a factor in migraine. In migraine, the most frequently used calcium channel blockers are verapamil and nimodipine.

Classic Migraine. See *Migraine with Aura*.

Cluster Headache. Type of vascular headache that occurs in a series or group of headaches. Cluster headaches occur more often in males. The headaches are characterized by their one-sided location, usually around one eye, and very brief duration, from a few minutes to one or two hours. The patient may experience several headaches per day for a period of one to several months.

Coexisting Migraine and Tension-type Headache. Also known as mixed headaches, chronic daily headache, and transformed migraine. These patients will report a history of two or more types of headaches occurring concurrently. Frequently, the patients will note a daily mild type of headache, similar to a tension-type headache, and a more severe headache, occurring several times in a week or a month, which resembles migraine. Patients with these headaches are prone to medication-habituation problems due to the frequency of their headaches. Often, they are also experiencing a concomitant depression.

Common Migraine. See *Migraine Without Aura*.

CT Scan. Computerized axial tomography (CT scan) uses a computer that merges many X rays from several angles into a single picture. The CT scan may be performed with or without a contrasting dye. If used to image the brain, the dye may be used to help identify a brain tumor or blood clot within the brain. CT scans of the brain are used frequently for headache patients to rule out an organic basis for their headaches.

Depression Headaches. These headaches are the most commonly occurring form of chronic tension-type headaches. In addition to daily or almost daily headaches, the patient will complain of a sleep disturbance in the form of frequent or early awakening. Often the patient does not outwardly appear to be depressed. Due to the frequency of the headaches, the patient may be prone to habituation problems with analgesics and barbiturates. The treatment of choice for these headaches are antidepressants, which are effective for their antidepressant action and possible analgesic effects.

Ergotamine. The ergotamine drugs are used to abort acute headaches. These drugs act on the blood vessels, preventing them from swelling. Ergotamine is available through prescription only and for administration in oral tablets, tablets for placement under the tongue, and as rectal suppositories. In order to avoid ergotamine rebound headaches, these drugs are never to be used on a daily basis.

Estrogen. Sex hormone produced in the ovary, placenta, testes, and possibly the adrenal glands. Estrogen is essential to the growth of the female sexual organs and also stimulates the secondary female characteristics, such as the development of full breasts and rounded hips. Estrogen levels vary within the menstrual cycle, rising dramatically from days nine to fourteen, about the time of ovulation, and then dropping dramatically from days twenty-four to twenty-eight, when menstrual flow begins. This decrease in estrogen levels is the impetus for the onset of menstrual migraine.

Histamine. A chemical that causes flushing, congestion, and tearing—all symptoms consistent with an allergic reaction.

Hormone. Hormones are the body's chemical messengers. They are produced by glands and are carried by the bloodstream to organs and tissues where they help regulate body systems such as growth, sexual development, metabolism, and the nervous system.

Menopause. The strictest definition of menopause is the final termination of the menstrual cycle. However, this stage in a woman's life may last for several years, as her menses changes and finally ends. Menopausal women may also experience a variety of symptoms, including hot flashes and fatigue.

Menstrual Migraine. This term refers to those migraine attacks associated with the menstrual cycle. Approximately 70 percent of female migraine sufferers will relate their headaches to their menses. Menstrual migraines are linked to changing levels of estrogen and progesterone. Headaches can occur immediately before menses, during the menstrual flow, or immediately after menses. Some patients may experience a migraine at the time of ovulation. The treatment of choice for menstrual migraine are the NSAIDs, starting two days before menses and continuing throughout the flow.

Migraine. Migraine is defined as a recurring headache that occurs one or more times per month and can last four to seventy-two hours. Typically, migraine is a one-sided headache, described as pounding or throbbing, and of moderate to incapacitating severity. Migraine is often termed a "sick" headache since it's associated with nausea, vomiting, and sensitivity to light. Some patients experience migraine with aura, with defined warning symptoms before the actual migraine attack (see *Aura*). The majority of patients with migraine do not experience the aura but may note a vague premonition of an impending migraine attack.

Migraine with Aura (Classic Migraine). Patients diagnosed with migraine with aura will have a history of an acute headache preceded by a neurological symptom, such as a visual disturbance (see *Aura*). The aura does not necessarily precede every migraine attack. Some elderly patients will note that the headaches have disappeared, but they are still troubled with symptoms of the aura.

Migraine Without Aura (Common Migraine). Patients with migraine without aura have never experienced the neurological warning signs of an aura. However, they may be able to predict an imminent headache by vague premonitory signs such as fatigue or burst of energy, increased or decreased appetite, or anxiety.

Monoamine Oxidase Inhibitors (MAOIs). The MAOIs are a form of antidepressant used as a second line of action in headaches related to depression. These drugs have also been shown effective in migraine treatment. Because these drugs are known to have severe interactions with foods containing tyramine and other vasoactive substances, patients on MAOIs must adhere to a tyramine-free diet. The MAOIs also interact with other medications, such as certain narcotics, over-the-counter cold remedies, and local anesthetics used in dental surgery. Patients must be carefully instructed regarding the precautions with the MAOIs.

MRI. Magnetic resonance imaging (MRI) is a technique that has revolutionized the evaluation of headache patients. By using a strong magnet, the physician is able to obtain thousands of views of the brain, and a computer blends these pictures to produce an astounding image of the brain. Unlike a CT scan, MRI can differentiate between normal and pathological tissues, and measure the density of the tissues. MRI can also detect problems at an early stage of the disease. Another advantage of MRI is that it can be performed without injecting a dye into the body and gives a clearer picture without the risks of CT scanning.

MSG. Monosodium glutamate (MSG) is used as a flavor enhancer in some foods, including processed meat, meat tenderizers, and Chinese cuisine. MSG can cause headaches and other symptoms in susceptible people within thirty minutes of ingesting the food item. Symptoms, besides headache, include sweating, chest tightness, and pressure over the face and chest. Migraine patients may be especially sensitive to foods containing MSG.

Nicotine. Nicotine is an essential substance in tobacco products, such as cigars and cigarettes. Because nicotine affects the blood vessels, smoking can contribute to the frequency and duration of migraine attacks. Patients with cluster headaches may often have to refrain from smoking during a series of headaches.

Nonsteroidal Anti-inflammatory Drugs (NSAIDs). These are a group of ever-expanding drugs that are known to be effective in a variety of chronic pain problems, including headaches. Aspirin is the original NSAID. It is believed that during a headache, a sterile inflammation occurs, and the headache will continue until the inflammation is resolved. The NSAIDs reduce this inflammation. The NSAIDs are the drugs of choice in the treatment of menstrual migraine. Examples of NSAIDs are ibuprofen, naproxen, naproxen sodium, fenoprofen calcium, and a host of others.

Oral Contraceptives. These drugs are used to prevent ovulation and therefore pregnancy. Birth control pills may contain estrogen or a combination of estrogen and progesterone. Oral contraceptives are known to increase the frequency, duration, severity, and complications of migraine.

OTC Medication. These are drugs that are available without a prescription. The best-known OTC is aspirin. Other OTC pain relievers used in headache are Tylenol, Advil, Motrin, Aleve, and Orudis.

PET Scanning. A scan using radioactive material to visualize the actual working of an organ like the brain. In other words, you are measuring the activity of an organ as opposed to viewing anatomy, as does MRI or CT scanning.

Prolactin. The pituitary hormone that controls lactation (breast milk production).

Prostaglandins. Fatty acids that act like hormones, and have good and bad functions. The bad functions can promote pain and headache; the good functions include their effects on the cardiovascular system, smooth muscle, and uterine contraction. If the prostaglandins are interrupted, the pain doesn't occur.

Scotoma. Scotoma is a form of aura in which the patient experiences a blind spot, of varying size, within the field of vision.

Serotonergic Drugs. Drugs that enhance or decrease the amount of serotonin and/or serotonin's actions.

Serotonin. Serotonin is a chemical substance similar to histamine that is most often found in the platelets. It is believed to be prominently involved in migraine attacks. Current headache research is directed to those agents that will block the receptors for serotonin. Sumatriptan is one of this class of drugs.

Spreading Depression. Lack of electrical activity in the brain.

Tension-type Headache. These headaches are thus called because emotional factors such as stress are believed to be their triggers. These headaches may be accompanied by pain in the neck and shoulders. They are caused by tightening of the muscles at the back of the neck and of the face and scalp. There are two types of tension-type headaches, episodic and chronic. The episodic form is easily controlled with over-the-counter analgesics. In the chronic form, the headaches occur on a daily or almost daily basis. In both forms, the headaches are two-sided and are often described as a tight band or a viselike ache. Chronic tension-type headaches can be due to anxiety or depression. Treatment of the acute headache should be limited to mild, nonhabituating analgesics. For prevention of the chronic form, the cause of the headaches must be determined. Chronic tension-type headaches due to anxiety are best treated with a mild tranquilizing agent, buspirone. For those headaches due to depression, the antidepressants are the drugs of choice in preventive treatment.

Triptans. These drugs affect the serotonin-like receptors, which play a role in migraine. These drugs have demonstrated beneficial results in migraine abortive therapy. Those currently available are sumatriptan, rizatriptan, naratriptan, and zolmitriptan.

Tyramine. Tyramine is a naturally occurring substance in certain foods. It is called vasoactive, as it can cause the blood vessels to expand and thus trigger a headache, such as migraine. Tyramine is found in a variety of foods, including aged cheese, nuts, yogurt, and is also found in alcoholic beverages. All headache patients should receive a tyramine-restricted diet to determine if avoiding these foods will decrease their headaches.

Vasoconstriction. Vasoconstriction refers to a decrease in the size of the blood vessels.

Vasodilation. Vasodilation refers to an increase in the size of the blood vessels.

Warnings of Migraine. These are vague symptoms that precede migraine without aura. They include fatigue or surge of energy, an increase or loss of appetite, restlessness, or listlessness.

APPENDIX

HEADACHE HISTORY

How many types of headache do you have? _____
_____

When did your headaches first start? _____
   How old were you when they started? _____
   Can you relate the start of your headache to any
   precipitating factor? _____
_____

Where is the headache located? _____
_____
_____

How often do you get the headaches? _____
_____
_____
_____

How severe are the headaches?_____
   Does it vary from headache to headache?_____
_____

How would you describe the pain? Is it throbbing, pulsing, pressure, tightness, etc.? _____

_____

Do you suffer from headaches after exertion, such as exercise, bending, stooping, lifting, straining? _____

_____

How long does your headache last? _____

   Does it vary in intensity throughout the day? _____

_____

Do you have any warning signs (seeing flashing light, halos, changes in vision) before the headache? _____

_____

Do you have any vague premonitions about the headache before it starts (fatigue or energy, increased or decreased appetite, quick temper, etc.)?_____

_____

Is your headache associated with any other complaint—nausea, vomiting, sensitivity to light or sound, nasal congestion, tearing, runny nose, neck pain, etc.? _____

_____

Do you have a sleep disturbance?_____

   Do you have difficulty falling asleep?_____

   Do you wake up often or early?_____

   Do you need an alarm clock?_____

Does anyone in your family have headaches (parents, siblings, grandparents, aunts, uncles, cousins)?_____
_____

For women: Do you notice any relationship between your headache and your periods?_____
    Did you have headaches during pregnancy?_____
    Are you on birth control pills or hormone-replacement therapy?_____

Do you notice an increase in headaches during certain times or seasons of the year?_____
    Do you have headaches at the holidays?_____
    Do you notice a change in headaches with changes in weather and altitude?_____

How would you describe your personality?_____
    Any problems at home, work, or school?_____
    _____

What tests have you had because of your headaches?_____
_____

Were you ever hospitalized for your headaches?_____
_____

Do you ever go to the emergency department for your headaches?_____
_____

What medications are you currently on for your headaches?

_____

How long does a bottle of aspirin or other over-the-counter pain reliever last?_____

_____

Are you on any other medications (not for headaches)?

_____

_____

Do you take over-the-counter remedies for your stomach or sinuses?_____

_____

Medical history:

_____

_____

Surgical history:

_____

_____

For women: How many pregnancies have you had?_____
   How many children?_____
   Have you ever been on birth control pills or hormone-
   replacement therapy? _____
   Are your periods regular?_____
   When was the first day of your last period?_____

Allergies/sensitivities:_____
  1. Drugs_____
  2. Foods_____
  3. Airborne_____

How many alcoholic beverages do you drink per week?

_____

Do you smoke?_____
  How many packs per day?_____

How many cups of coffee/tea/cola beverages do you consume
per day?_____

_____

Drug History *(for headaches)*

Name _____   Date _____

Name of drug (dose)	How long did you take drug?	Did it help?	If discontinued, why?

Previous Consultations with Physicians

Name(s) of Physician(s) _____ Date _____

1. _____
2. _____
3. _____
4. _____
5. _____
6. _____

Previous Hospitalizations *(for headaches)*

Name(s) of Physician(s) _____ Date _____

1. _____
2. _____
3. _____
4. _____
5. _____
6. _____

Previous Emergency Department Visits *(due to headaches)*

Name(s) of Physician(s): _____ Date_____

1. _____

2. _____

3. _____

4. _____

5. _____

6. _____

HEADACHE CALENDAR

Patient's Name: _____

Date	Time Onset Ending (record hour and A.M./P.M.)		(1) Severity of Headache	(2) Psychic and Physical Factors	(3) Food and Drink Excesses	Medication Taken and Dosage	(4) Relief of Headache

Headache Keys

(1) Severity Scale

1		5		10
None	Mild		Moderate	Severe

(2) Psychic and Physical Factors

1. Emotional upset/family or friends
2. Emotional upset/occupation
3. Business/reversal
4. Business/success
5. Vacation days
6. Weekends
7. Strenuous exercise
8. Strenuous labor
9. High-altitude location
10. Anticipation anxiety
11. Crisis/serious
12. Post-crisis period
13. New job/position
14. New move
15. Menstrual days
16. Physical illness
17. Oversleeping
18. Weather
19. Fasting
20. Missing a meal
21. Other_____

(3) Relief Scale

1		5		10
Complete	Moderate		Mild	No Relief

(4) Food and Drink Excesses

A. Ripened cheeses (pizza)
B. Herring
C. Chocolate
D. Vinegar
E. Fermented foods (pickled or marinated sour cream/yogurt)
F. Freshly baked yeast products
G. Nuts (peanut butter)
H. Monosodium glutamate (MSG—Chinese food)
I. Pods of broad beans
J. Onions
K. Canned figs
L. Citrus foods
M. Bananas
N. Pork
O. Caffeinated beverages (cola)
P. Avocado
Q. Fermented sausage (cured cold cuts)
R. Chicken livers
S. Wine
T. Alcohol
U. Beer

(Patients on Nardil and/or Marplan should follow the original diet given them)

INDEX

ABOUT THE AUTHORS

Seymour Diamond, M.D., an internationally recognized expert in management of headache pain, is the founder and director of the Diamond Headache Clinic in Chicago, Illinois, the oldest and largest private clinic in the United States devoted solely to headache. The author of *The Hormone Headache* and the coeditor of *The Practicing Physician's Approach to Headache*, Dr. Diamond has contributed to twenty other headache books and has written more than three hundred articles on the subject of headache.

Mary A. Franklin has been a member of the nursing and administrative staffs at the Diamond Headache Clinic since 1970. She is currently the clinic's vice president of Publishing and Administration and has been the managing editor of *Headache Quarterly: Current Treatment and Research* since its inception in 1990.